NO MORE
HEARTBURN

NO MORE HEARTBURN

Stop the Pain in 30 Days—Naturally!

The Safe, Effective Way
to Prevent and Heal Chronic
Gastrointestinal Disorders

SHERRY A. ROGERS, M.D.

KENSINGTON BOOKS
http://www.kensingtonbooks.com

This book is designed to provide accurate and authoritative information in regard to the subject matter covered. It is sold with the understanding that the publisher is not engaged in rendering medical or related professional services and that without personal consultation the author cannot and does not render judgment or advice about a particular patient or medical condition. If medical advice is required, the services of a competent professional should be sought. While every attempt has been made to provide accurate information, the author and publisher cannot be held responsible for any errors or omissions.

KENSINGTON BOOKS are published by

Kensington Publishing Corp.
850 Third Avenue
New York, NY 10022

ISBN 1-57566-510-7

First Printing: February, 2000
20 19 18 17 16 15 14 13

Printed in the United States of America

Not only this book, but my whole life is dedicated to Luscious, who after thirty years is still God's greatest gift to me.

Contents

Chapter 3: Curing the Most Commonly Missed Cause of Gut Disease 51

Introduction

Why do we need a book on banishing heartburn? We already know how to spell relief: R-O-L-A-I-D-S—or Maalox, Mylanta, or Di-Gel. If those fail, there are the great acid inhibitors that went from prescription to over-the-counter status all too quickly like Pepcid, Zantac, Tagamet, and Axid. And if those fail to give relief, there is a whole new generation of proton-pump inhibitors emerging, like Prilosec and Prevacid, as well as other potent prescription medications that squelch possible symptoms.

As a recent *New England Journal of Medicine* article (Lagergren) by specialists at the prestigious Karolinska Institute in Stockholm have reported, *heartburn is anything but harmless.* In fact, it carries a high risk of evolving into cancer of the esophagus, for which there is still no cure. And this heightened risk for esophageal cancer is not double or triple, but forty-three times that of those who do not suffer from heartburn or indigestion! Esophageal cancer is so vicious that fewer than twelve people out of one hundred live to five years after diagnosis. In just the last two decades, the number of esophageal cancer victims each year has increased eightfold, making it the fastest growing cancer nationwide.

Add to this an even more important fact that has emerged from the research: getting medical treatment for heartburn increases, not lessens, your chances of getting cancer. Be that as it may, gastroenterologists at noted medical schools still recommend that patients take their medications "continuously and indefinitely" (Cohen).

Why? Because drugs are the major tools of modern medicine. For example, many doctors view symptoms as a deficiency of drugs, either because the drugs have failed to treat the symptoms or because they have actually caused the symptoms. In response, these same doctors go on to prescribe more, if different, drugs, even though studies are now showing that such treatments can actually increase one's chances of getting cancer.

Traditional medicine remains bewildered about why people who receive the best treatment that doctors can offer do worse than those who are not treated. At the same time, doctors seem powerless as they watch the evolution from heartburn to X ray-diagnosed reflux, to biopsied Barrett's esophagus, to fulminant cancer, knowing all the while that the uncontrollable cancerous transformation may actually be quickened by medical treatment.

When drugs fail completely, traditional medicine resorts to surgery. Now, the standard treatment for this transition stage (called Barrett's esophagus) from reflux or heartburn to cancer is to laser or burn abnormal precancerous cells. But the burning of precancerous cells, like medications, does nothing to identify and correct the underlying cause. Instead, physicians watch and wait, seemingly helpless to abort the progression to full-blown cancer.

With one in five people suffering from heartburn and indigestion and another one in five suffering from irritable bowel syndrome (IBS) or spastic colitis, is it any wonder that drugs that calm the gut are always among the top ten prescription and nonprescription medications sold nationwide? Furthermore, when studies appear like the one from Stockholm (noted above) which show an acceleration in the progression to cancer by virtue of medication use, is it any wonder that esophageal and other cancers have escalated to the number two cause of death in the United States alone?

Why should something as seemingly harmless as indigestion progress to cancer? Perhaps the modus operandi in medicine is to blame. Medicating rather than educating patients about how to find the real cause(s) of their condition(s) and thereby freeing themselves of medications and symptoms causes the circle to close in on itself. Although you can see your family doctor, be referred to the gut specialist (gastroenterologist), or surf the Net for instructions on how to rid yourself of symptoms, be medication-free and avoid a progression to cancer, chances are slim to none that you will find the answers you need. I have written this book so that you and those you care for can understand why you suffer and how to correct the cause(s) of symptoms once and for all.

Yes, the absurdity of the current medical system sometimes borders on the unbelievable as physicians, pharmaceutical companies and insurance companies desperately cling to their belief in drugs as the panacea for each and every condition, even when their own studies contradict them. Nor is this the only example of the illogical nature of traditional medicine today.

For instance, a common cause of indigestion, ulcers, and eventual stomach cancer is the bacteria that thrive in city water supplies. Years ago researchers began treating gastritis, heartburn, and indigestion resulting from this bacteria with H2–blockers like Zantac and Pepcid. They quickly found that these drugs, while making the stomach feel better, did not cure the problem. As soon as people stopped taking the drug, their symptoms recurred. And the longer folks were on acid inhibitors, the worse the stomach bug grew, even so far as to trigger cancer, this time of the stomach and the duodenum.

Even worse, researchers found that within a twelve-month period over half the folks on H2–blockers (sixty-one out of one hundred patients) had destroyed their stomach linings (Zucca). Atrophic gastritis, this destruction of the stomach lining, can also lead to malnutrition and its associated effects, senility, and cancer. Yes, the *sick get sicker, quicker,* when drugs are used to mask symptoms without searching for causes. Fortunately, you can learn how to find the cause or causes of your symptom(s) right here in this book.

Ironically, despite research showing that the acid-squelcher Prilosec makes the ulcer-causing stomach bug trigger cancer of the stomach more quickly, current treatment recommendations for heartburn include not one, but two antibiotics plus Prilosec! Bear in mind that Prilosec wipes out the body's natural defenses against the bug—the stomach acid—allowing the bug to grow even more viciously. The bug can do either of two things: trigger cancer or rot out the stomach lining with atrophic gastritis.

In addition, the antibiotics commonly prescribed for this stomach bug, by causing yeast or fungus overgrowth in the gut, can also trigger a mountain of other conditions that seem unrelated, including lupus, multiple sclerosis, thyroiditis, chronic fatigue, depression, fibromyalgia, rheumatoid arthritis, chronic prostatitis, chemical sensitivity, food allergies, brain fog, cancer, and many more.

Unfortunately, gut torture doesn't end here, as anyone with ulcerative colitis or Crohn's disease can attest. True to form, these victims, after years of drugs, hospitalizations, even emergency transfusions, often end up undergoing a colectomy and colostomy, and having to wear a bag glued to the abdominal wall to collect stool as the nagging threat of cancer still hovers overhead. But remember, whether your problem begins in the mouth with recurrent canker sores and mouth ulcers, or reaches to the opposite end of the gut with rectal itching and bleeding, there is a cause for it.

Or perhaps your gut is the least of your problems and you hardly give a thought to a little gas, bloating, or indigestion. You may have much bigger problems that no one can solve, or that, as you've been told, you must learn to live with. Conditions such as leaky gut syndrome (LGS, or intestinal hyperpermeability) and chronic Candida intestinalis (overgrowth of yeast from antibiotics or sweets, for example) are just a few of the major reasons why many folks are at a standstill.

Regardless of how remote from the gut their diagnostic label is, these conditions will never get better until the gut is healed. But since an ill gut presents common to no symptoms at all, folks never dream that the gut is holding them back from ever healing completely. It matters not if you are diagnosed with high cholesterol, migraines, arthritis, or cancer. If the gut is not completely healthy, then you have nary a hope of completely healing any other condition in the body.

If you are among those who suffer from symptoms in the gut—over a third of the population—you have two choices: (1) You can suppress the symptoms with drugs while the underlying causes progress to cancer or other illnesses. (2) Or you can learn how to find the causes and cures in your search for a drug-free, symptom-free life. Some of the solutions are ridiculously logical and simple. Whether your solutions come easily or require more detailed instruction, I guide you along each step of the way. For once you possess the power to heal yourself, no one can ever take it away from you. As I have told patients from all over the world during three decades of medical practice, I have three goals:

1. to help you get rid of your symptoms
2. to help you get rid of your drugs
3. to help you get rid of me.

When I can do all that, I have done my job as a physician and teacher. I have empowered you with knowledge that will serve you for the rest of your life.

CHAPTER 1

How Standard Medical Treatments Guarantee That the Sick Will Get Sicker, Quicker

It would be difficult to watch a few hours of television and not be convinced that, by taking this or that drug, your gut problems are over. You might even be advised to take something before you leave your house for some imprudent eating. The sad part is that, despite being wonderfully effective in providing fast relief, taking the gastrointestinal drugs advertised on TV only guarantees that your condition will get worse.

You Are Not Alone

Although gut symptoms may not be a topic for polite conversation, they are among the top ten symptoms that bring folks to the doctor. In fact, one out of every four patients has a complaint of something wrong with his or her intestinal tract. Indeed, researchers have found that over a three-month period, seven out of ten households experience some sort of gastrointestinal symptoms and miss three times as many days a year from work as those without gut symptoms (Drossman). Other researchers offer corroborating evidence, with at least four out of ten folks experiencing indigestion (Jones). And when such folks go to a clinic, their doctors are unable to find any cause for their symptoms in over half of these cases (Johannessen).

If you still think that you are in the minority, look at the pharmacy shelves brimming with medications for calming the gut, sopping up acid, turning off acid, relieving heartburn and indigestion, and easing constipation, and the millions of advertising dollars spent on them each year. Did you know that the top-selling gut drug stops the production of stomach acid, the very acid you need to ensure the digestion and absorption of the foods and liquids you consume?

No, you are not alone.

"You'll Just Have to Learn to Live with It"

Unfortunately, the two leading diagnoses for stomach and gut complaints are not ulcers or cancer, but dyspepsia and irritable bowel syndrome (IBS). Do these fancy terms mean anything more than this to your doctor: "I haven't the foggiest notion of what is causing your symptoms. But I do have a large assortment of drugs that will calm and mask your symptoms— drugs you can take for the rest of your life. You'll just have to learn to live with it."

I, for one, do not think so.

The fact is that gastrointestinal specialists do not know how to find the causes of, or the cures for, the top two diseases they encounter each day of their careers in clinical practice. Much less do they find the curable causes for other, more serious gut diseases like Crohn's disease or gastrointestinal cancers.

Fortunately, when you've finished reading this book you should know more about finding the causes of and cures for most intestinal symptoms than the majority of the world's gut specialists. How do I know this? Because of the more than thirty years of successes my medical colleagues and I have had. There are thousands of patients who, having been told "There's nothing you can do for this condition," or "You'll just have to learn to live with it," or "You'll need to take medication to control symptoms for the rest of your life," have proven their specialists wrong. They have used the techniques you are about to learn to find the causes of and cures for their symptoms.

Are you ready for one of the most important adventures of your life? What could be more invigorating than learning how to control your health? Regardless of your symptoms or disease, health begins in the gut. If the gut is not healthy, then how can any other organ heal? And if you already know you have gut symptoms, then you have only one real choice before you—to find the cause and heal it once and for all.

Medications Turn Off the Gut's
Only Means of Communication

How does your intestinal tract tell you something is wrong? Nausea, heartburn, acid indigestion, excessive intestinal gas and bloating, uncontrollable burping, cramps, diarrhea, constipation, blood and mucus—that's how. These are the only ways your gut can tell you that if you don't find and fix what's broken, your problems will only worsen.

The gastrointestinal (GI) tract involves everything from the mouth to the rectum, including the digestive juices from the mouth's salivary glands, the esophagus (the tube connecting the mouth to the stomach), the small intestine (where most food absorption occurs), and the large intestine (where reabsorption or conservation of water and other nutrients occurs). Because secretions crucial to GI tract function involve bile (stored in the gall bladder which is tucked up beneath the liver), as well as lipase and amylase from the pancreas (which is nestled behind the stomach), these are included here as well.

The standard medical workup for chronic gas, bloating, and indigestion consists of a history; a physical; X rays of the gut; and scoping of the gut, beginning with esophagoscopy, gastroscopy, and even duodenoscopy. A more extensive search can reach into the other end with a sigmoidoscopy or further up, as far as the junction between the large and small intestines, with a colonoscopy.

When everything seems or looks normal, a diagnosis of IBS or irritable bowel disease or inflammatory bowel disease (IBD) is made. Again, such diagnoses usually boil down to the same thing for doctors, who use the terminology to mask the fact that they simply don't know why chronic gas, bloating, and indigestion occurs. Such diagnoses also help to prevent the gastroenterologist, or gut specialist, from using all the techniques that you will learn about here, and which will enable and empower you to uncover the real causes.

Then, too, there are vast limitations to the standard battery of medical tests. First, they do not tell how well you are digesting your food, how effectively you are absorbing nutrients, or even if you cannot absorb food at all—a condition known as overt malabsorption. The standard tests also fail to evaluate your digestive functions as a whole.

For example, did you know that digestion begins in the eyes, nose, ears, and brain, and that how you sense and think about food affects how you digest it? Furthermore, if you eat under stressful conditions, you will be mired in indigestion despite the doctor's X rays and scopes. As the bolus of food sits in your stomach, unable to move along to the small intestine, it will ferment and decay. Noxious gasses will rise to the esophagus and cause belching and foul breath.

In time, as the bolus of food and ballooning gasses distend the esophagus, the one protective valve between the stomach and esophagus will stretch and leak. Gases now trapped in the esophagus will give that familiar retrosternal (behind the breastbone) agony of heartburn. Add to that the backflow of undigested food mixed with sharply irritating stomach acids and your pain may increase to the point where breathing becomes difficult.

As this fermenting and decaying mass slides slowly along the gut, you can suffer more abdominal bloating and painful cramps and, eventually, alternating dirrahea and constipation. Again, however, because the standard tests will not show evidence of pathology here, you will be given a clean bill of health.

Furthermore, the tests that gastroenterologists perform ignore function and tend to focus on lesions (like ulcers), colitis, or cancers. But as the brief review of secretions from the GI tract below shows, the gut is a highly integrated system. Indeed, despite the fact that health depends on the synergistic action of gut and GI tract secretions, the first goal of modern medicine is to turn off some or all of them. In an already ailing system, that is the last thing you should do. Turning off what remaining functions exist, and doing so without question as to reason or purpose, is very much like throwing gasoline on a smoldering fire. The result? An eventual blaze of other, seemingly unrelated diseases.

As a starter for understanding indigestion, consider this: We Americans eat the largest variety of foods in the world, which strains our digestive capacity. As the original hunter-gatherer, homo sapiens rarely found such a banquet for every meal in the wild. On top of this, we Americans eat the most processed, chemicalized and difficult to digest food in the world. Adding insult to injury, with modern antacids we sop up what little digestive acid there is, axing the already deficient digestive and bug-killing capacities of our stomachs. When you think of what we ask the digestive system to do every day, it appears to be a pretty awesome piece of equipment. But as you will learn, the gut has another function infinitely more important than digestion.

We might naively think that after a few chews, a swallow, and several hours' time, the digestion of foods and liquids ends. But digestion is a complicated process that depends on many factors. For example, a journey down the gut involves contact with dozens of digestive enzymes. Let's take a peek at where they orginate, in what secretions, and what they do. (See Table 1.)

Let's now take a look at how some of the more common gut medications affect the complicated process of digestion. You should know that, as a physician, it was an eye-opener for me when I discovered that the common gut medications eventually worsen the conditions they were developed for.

Table 1. The Sources and Functions of our Many Digestive Enzymes

Organ	Secretion	Function/Digestion
Brain	neurotransmitters, V.I.P.	Promotes parasympathetic relaxation of the gut and secretion of digestive juices
Mouth	salivary amylase	starches
	lingual lipase	triglycerides
Teeth		break down food
Stomach	pepsin	proteins
	gastric lipase	triglycerides
Pancreas	trypsin	proteins
	chymotrypsin	proteins
	elastase	elastin
	carboxypeptidase	proteins
	colipase	fat
	pancreatic lipase	
	cholesteryl ester hydrolase	cholesteryl esters
	amylase	starch
	ribonuclease (RNA)	
	deoxyribonuclease (DNA)	
	phospholipase	fatty acids
intestinal mucosa	enteropeptidase	activates trypsinogen
	aminopeptidase	peptides
	dipeptidases	dipeptides
	glucoamylase	maltose
	lactase	lactose (milk sugar)
	sucrase	sucrose (table sugar)
	dextrinase	dextrins
	nuclease	nucleic acids
	peptidases	peptides

Source: Ganong WF. *Review of Medical Physiology,* 5th ed. Norwalk, CT: Appleton & Lange, 1991, p. 438.

I was trained to rely on and trust in drugs. Now that the mass marketing of drugs has reached the consumer, you, too, will be led down the same thorny path. I'm here to see that that does not happen.

"My Doctor Said, 'Mylanta'"

The commercial that boasted instantaneous relief from symptoms with Mylanta created a spectrum of problems that I began to see in my practice more and more. Quite simply, as Mylanta sopped up the acid that prompts indigestion, it also depleted the same acid we need for absorbing minerals. Without a sufficient quantity of minerals we are vulnerable to many diseases, from depression to cancer. Also, antacids often contain aluminum, which, as it collects in the brain, contributes to early senility and memory loss. At the same time, by taking antacids to relieve symptoms, you can all too easily ignore the real cause of your distress, or even the need to uncover it. Unfortunately, the resulting false sense of security is dangerous.

Is it any wonder then that the third-most-common cause of death in the United States, after arteriosclerosis (heart attacks and strokes) and cancer, is drug reactions? There is a veritable epidemic of drug-induced diseases. In this regard, your continued use of antacids is foolish. When you come to understand why, you'll also know how to uncover the cause of your indigestion and what steps to take to resolve it heathfully.

Even a seemingly harmless antacid like Mylanta can cause serious symptoms. For example, I know two surgeons who treated their own "heartburn" with Mylanta for over a month before they required emergency heart surgery. In other words, their diagnosis was wrong! They had life-threatening angina that they mistakenly thought was heartburn.

Another man treated his ulcer symptoms with Mylanta for years and spent a fortune on the psychiatrist's couch for depression. Thankfully, once I medically removed the aluminum that had accumulated in his brain from the antacids, his depression cleared and he was able to throw away the antidepressants that left him feeling like a zombie.

Scientists have known for over two decades that the aluminum left over from the consumption of antacids (Kaehny) finally accumulates in brain enzymes. There, the aluminum wreaks havoc (Banks), shriveling the brain structure into a nonfunctioning, tangled mess (Perl 1980, 1990), which scientists rightly call "neurofibrillary tangles." Fortunately, if the problem is suspected early enough, it can be diagnosed and reversed. (See Chapter 6.)

One patient of mine, Agnes, frequently abused her stomach with greasy fried foods and processed fast foods that she knew disagreed with her. She also knew that a swig of antacid would bring relief. What she did not know was that the antacid sopped up the gastric acid she needed to absorb priceless minerals like calcium. She ended up with osteoporosis and a hip fracture.

The magnesium levels of another patient, Art, became so depleted from antacids that inhibited his mineral absorption that his back went into violent spasm where an old ruptured disc was. Not knowing any better, he had surgery, but afterward still had back spasms—until his magnesium deficiency was diagnosed and treated. Art was lucky; Stan, another patient, was not. From inhibiting the absorption of his minerals with antacids, Stan suffered a sudden, fatal cardiac arrest.

If you prefer Tums-type antacids because they also give you calcium, consider again. If all that calcium carbonate is sopping up or neutralizing gastric acid, where does the acid necessary to ionize the calcium for absorption later on down the digestive tract come from? It is somewhat illogical to believe that much calcium can be absorbed when you shut down the acid-promoting phase needed for the absorption of calcium and other minerals in general.

Gastroesophageal reflux disease (GERD) is another popular diagnosis that folks take antacids for. With GERD, the valve between the esophagus and stomach suddenly becomes defective. In response, doctors commonly prescribe drugs to turn off the stomach's acid secretion, and then more drugs to hurry the emptying of the stomach. If all else fails, you can have surgery to tighten the defective valve. Nonetheless, if this is a physical defect, why does it appear when it does, at this particular stage of your life?

I always like to step back to find out why a structure like the gastroesophageal valve, a valve that served you in good stead for so many years, suddenly gives out. What would cause the valve to allow stomach acid to backtrack or reflux into the esophagus?

One major cause here is the way Americans tend to eat: rushed meals and poor chewing, large meals, with many different types of foods, processed foods with difficult-to-digest artificial ingredients, often accompanied by large amounts of liquid that dilute the already-compromised digestive juices. Large, undigestible meals stretch the stomach and its valve beyond capacity. As a result, the valve does not close properly and the poorly digested food backs up, irritating the GI tract. Chronic irritation here all too easily develops into esophagitis, hiatus hernia, heartburn, or indigestion. But all, regardless of label, can be corrected without surgery in the vast majority of cases.

The moral of the story is clear: When you use medications to suppress or to hide symptoms, and so avoid finding the true cause, you pay three hefty prices:

1. shutting down or turning off a normal physiologic function of the body
2. ignoring the cause of the original problem, so that it continues to worsen
3. the drugs' numerous side effects.

When you take antacids, you miss a wonderful chance to find out and fix what's wrong before it gets worse. In addition, you suffer from the side effects of antacids, including aluminum toxicity, which damages brain tissue, along with an inhibition of the body's natural capacity to absorb the priceless minerals that health hinges on. Have no fear though. You will find out why the gastroesophageal valve becomes defective at any stage of life and how to avoid surgery intended to fix it.

The Tagamet Tragedy

Why is Tagamet (generic name, cimetidine) so popular now? That's easy: As soon as its patent expired, it became available over the counter and, with a TV ad campaign to espouse its virtues, sales skyrocketed. Tagamet, however, is different from its older antacid relatives. It does not just sop up acid; it blocks the H2 acid-secretion site on the stomach cells so that they do not release gastric juices. Though this makes Tagamet more effective, it also increases the side effects exponentially.

For example, on October 14, 1991, an article appeared in the *Wall Street Journal* about Mr. Latimer, a vigorous, athletic, 36-year-old Dallas-based petroleum engineer whose life, as he knew it, stopped one Saturday as he mowed his newly pesticided lawn. Suddenly, something was very wrong— he was overcome by dizzness, nausea, chest tightness, runny nose, and a pounding headache. Over the next several months these and newer symptoms, like an uncontrollable jerking of the eyes, worsened. In less than half a year, he was diagnosed with testicular cancer, and his health continued to go downhill.

Six years later, his health had deteriorated even more. He was exhausted, and had such neuromuscular problems that he couldn't even ride a bike, had difficulty walking, and had frequent seizures. A toxicologist, three neurologists, and two neuro-ophthalmologists independently agreed that he had organophosphate pesticide poisoning. Unfortunately, his vulnerability to the poisoning increased by virtue of his daily consumption of 900 milligrams of Tagamet, which grossly interfered with his ability to detoxify the common pesticide, diazinon. As a result the diazinon accumulated in his body, triggering cancer, exacerbating his chronic fatigue, and causing a disabling neurological poisoning complete with seizures and peculiar nightmares that left over half a dozen physicians powerless.

Because he was taking the H2-blocker Tagamet, which vied for the same detoxification pathways in his body as the pesticide did, he did not have enough detoxification reserve. Consequently, the pesticide's carcinogenic properties were magnified, not detoxified. Further undetoxified pesticide residues damaged his mitochondria, the delicate little organelles inside each cell where energy is made, causing chronic fatigue. And they continued to damage his nervous system, especially the brain.

The fact that Tagamet and similar H2-blockers vie for the same detoxification enzymes is common knowledge in medicine. Even the *Physicians' Desk Reference (PDR)*, the standard textbook that describes drug actions and side effects, warns that Tagamet-like drugs compromise detoxification pathways. Another problem concerns our individual biochemistry. There is no way to know with exactitude how H2-blockers will affect each person. Add to this our daily exposures to toxic substances at home, work, in traffic, in- and outdoors, and in food and water, all of which must be detoxified, and our weaknesses grow. One thing is quite clear though: If the detoxification enzymes are slowed down by Tagamet, then symptoms and side effects from these exposures can be exacerbated. It's also important not to overlook the many other drugs a person may be taking, whether self- or physician-prescribed. An undue combination of drugs may greatly magnify undesired effects.

As sick as he was, Mr. Latimer was still fortunate. He did not suffer from all the possible side effects of Tagamet, which include cardiac arrhythmia, hypertension, gynecomastia or breast enlargement in men, headaches, dizziness, low white-blood-cell count, and heart block. Such side effects can occur at any time, even years after initially taking the drug, which decreases the likelihood of your associating the appearance of symptoms with the drug.

And get this: The drug you are taking for GI symptoms can also cause diarrhea. Yes, diarrhea is a side effect of Tagamet and all related drugs. Finally, it is important for you to remember that if you are taking Tagamet or other similar drugs, like Zantac (ranitidine), Axid (nizatidine), Pepcid (famotidine), or Mylanta AR Acid Reducer (famotidine), they also interfere with your body's ability to detoxify the poisons you consume on a daily basis.

Here's another side effect of Tagamet and other H2-blockers: They can make one alcoholic drink seem like two or more (Leiber). For example, researchers found that when study subjects took Zantac or Tagamet before imbibing alcohol, their blood alcohol levels increased 34 to 92 percent higher than normal. Such an increase in blood alcohol levels could bring disastrous results for the unsuspecting person who listens to popular TV commercials and premedicates before making a dietary indiscretion that includes alcohol. Unfortunately, the commercials don't also warn that he or she might also triple his or her chances of having a fatal auto accident on the way home from the party.

The triple moral of this story is: (1) the more precise the nature of the medication in turning off normal bodily functions, the more secondary damage it is capable of; (2) all systemic medicines (those that go into the entire body or system) exert their chemistry on every cell of the body, despite the fact that they are designed to turn off the function of only one particular area, so they have far-reaching effects; and (3) every systemic medicine uses up detoxification pathways in order to be detoxified or metabolized itself.

The Prilosec/Prevacid Scam

Prilosec (generic name, omeprazole) has led the pack in terms of advertising for prescription drugs. The Sunday paper in nearly every U.S. city has sported full-page ads expounding Prilosec's acid-inhibiting nature, but not its side effects. Its side effects include diarrhea, abdominal pain, nausea, vomiting, gas, constipation, acid reflux, and carcinoid tumors in the gut.

But it doesn't stop there. Prilosec can cause fatal liver rot (necrosis), fatal pancreatitis, headache, back pain, hair loss, toxic epidermal necrolysis (a condition where your skin becomes red and scaly, then finally, painfully oozes and peels off), or it can stop the production of blood cells. There are other side effects, but I don't want to scare you. Like Tagamet, Prilosec can severely distort or compromise the detoxification of other drugs.

But Prilosec and similar drugs, which include Prevacid (lansoprazole), reach even further into the workings of the cell to stop normal function than Tagamet does. As proton-pump inhibitors, Prilosec-type drugs stop the stomach cells from producing acid altogether. Prilosec-type drugs essentially curtail normal stomach function, highlighting again what seems now a golden rule in medicine: If something is malfunctioning, make it malfunction even more, at least enough to mask the initial symptom.

Proton-pump inhitors can also turn off other important stomach functions, especially those that require healthy parietal cells in the stomach lining, which are responsible for the secretion of intrinsic factor. Why is this important? Because without it you can't absorb vitamin B_{12}. And when you slow down the absorption of B_{12}, you set yourself up for all sorts of symptoms from accelerated arteriosclerosis, depression, or fatigue to undiagnosable numbness, tingling, and other nerve dysfunctions. Then, if you happen to be a person with chronic disease, like diabetes or arteriosclerosis, you accelerate the side effects of that disease. Early aging, cataracts, painful neuropathy, even early death from heart attack, and more are only some of the side effects you may encounter.

Yes, the further you reach into a cell to distort its basic actions, the more dangerous the side effects become—and the sick get sicker, quicker. With Prilosec-type drugs you are shutting down the basic function of the stomach cell, which is to secrete acid to digest your food. Remember, some of the many functions of stomach acid include killing fungi, viruses, and bacteria to provide a medium for initiating the absorption of minerals, digestion of food, and regulation of body acid/base, or pH, balance –functions we need to stay healthy.

For its part, Prevacid has a fluoride molecule sitting in it which gives it an extra toxicity, and perhaps accounts for the higher rate of reported tumors in those who use it. Did you know that folks living in areas with fluorinated water experience higher rates of some cancers and higher death rates than folks who live elsewhere (Kohn, Erikson)?

CASE HISTORY

"I really blew it this time," Hank admitted sheepishly. "I know how you're always warning us about not getting on the medication merry-go-round; that once you start taking one drug, you suddenly need a whole slew of them. Well, I've got a pocket full of pills and a stable full of specialists—and I've never felt lousier!"

After I took a special environmental medicine history and did tests that none of his specialists had ever heard of (Chapter 7), we pieced together the scenario of Hank's downfall and progressively returned him back to better health.

It all started when he overindulged in sweets during the holidays and then didn't nip the habit in the bud. Because his immune system had been weakened by the paralyzing effect that sugar has on white blood cells, he got a sinus infection. After taking the antibiotics that his doctor prescribed, the yeast in his stomach overgrew to the point of causing gnawing pain. The doctor then ordered X rays to determine what was wrong, but the X rays revealed nothing. And how could they? X rays can show ulcers but not yeast overgrowth. The doctor then put Hank on Prilosec, the current treatment for reducing acid production in the stomach. Because no one looked for the yeast and since Prilosec is so effective at turning off acid secretion, which normally controls invading yeast, the Candida burgeoned.

As long as Hank took the Prilosec, his stomach didn't bother him all that much, but within six months his blood pressure was up. A diuretic, or fluid pill, controlled the rise in his blood pressure, but it lowered his magnesium level, which was, by virtue of the Prilosec, already low.

Within a few more months, Hank had unknowingly tripled his loss of magnesium: the Prilosec and the diuretic for his blood pressure enhanced the magnesium loss, which further irritated his stomach. At the same time, he developed a cardiac arrhythmia, perhaps caused by his magnesium loss. At this point his doctor was stumped and referred Hank to another specialist. He was simply too young for atrial fibrillation, but there it was nonetheless. The specialist prescribed another drug, a calcium-channel blocker, to treat the cardiac arrhthmia. Although commonly prescribed by cardiologists, calcium-channel blockers carry a multitude of side effects, including a near doubling of cancer and heart attach rates as well as being causative in senile deterioration of the brain.

Hank realized he had let things slide too far when, within a year, he had hired a gastroenterologist, was on a first-name basis with a cardiologist, and his doctor, who had just done a physical on him, told him he looked great.

When Hank finally came to me, I understood his malaise immediately. First I ordered a special study of his stool that revealed the Candida overgrowth plus another bug, klebsiella. A mineral assay of his blood revealed magnesium, as well as manganese, selenium, and chromium deficiencies. When we killed the abnormal stomach bugs and corrected his mineral deficiencies, Hank's symptoms melted away and he no longer required drugs. In addition, the other side effects he had acquired from his previous drug regimen—like his inability to have an erection, unwarranted depression, and mysterious fatigue—all disappeared. That is what environmental functional medicine is all about. Finding the cause and getting rid of a life sentence of drugs.

Propulcid, Cytotec, Actigall , Carafate, and Over-the-Counter Medications

Propulsid (cisapride), another type of prescription drug used mostly for diabetics and others with poor nerve-muscle tone, also affects the GI tract. By enhancing the release of acetylcholine, the main nerve-to-muscle transmitter, Propulsid accelerates gastric emptying. More specifically, Propulsid strengthens the chemical that allows nerves to prompt muscle contraction, hurrying food through the gut, thereby relieving heartburn and reflux in some cases. Reglan (metoclopramide) is another brand of the same family.

When you tamper with nerve function, however, you can affect other areas of the body. With Propulcid, side effects include serious electrocardiogram (EKG) abnormalities, causing rhythm disturbances like potentially fatal ventricular tachycardia and ventricular fibrillation, as well as headache, diarrhea, abdominal pain, nausea, constipation, anxiety, arthralgia (joint pain), myalgia (aching all over), and more.

Then there is the category of prostaglandin analogues, or cytoprotective, drugs. Cytotec (misprostol), for example, is designed to protect the stomach from ulcers produced by the nonsteroidal anti-inflammatory drugs (NSAIDs) for arthritis, like ibuprofen, Aleve, Advil, Motrin, Naprosyn, and others. It not only inhibits the production of stomach acid, but also that of another digestive juice, pepsin, while increasing alkaline bicarbonate and mucus production. It does not work further down the gut to prevent duodenal ulcers, however.

Cytotec has the usual long list of gut side effects, since it does nothing to actually fix what is broken, but merely masks it. These include diarrhea, abdominal pain, nausea, gas, headache, heartburn, vomiting, and constipation. But a drug that powerful can do other nasty things in the body with additional side effects such as high blood pressure, body aches, chest pain, heart arrhythmia, impotence, fever, blood clots, intestinal hemorrhaging, abnormal menses, and uterine cramps; it has been shown to induce abortion.

There are even more specialized prescription medications, like Actigall, to dissolve gallstones, but again side effects make it worth your while to consider learning the gall bladder flush. (See Chapter 6 or you can refer to my previous book *Wellness Against All Odds.*)

Carafate (sucralfate) is a medication designed to coat duodenal and gastric ulcers to protect them from painful stomach acid. Theoretically, patients would use the drug for only a short while to help heal an ulcer. But as you will learn in the next chapters, since doctors rarely look for the cause of the ulcer, folks end up taking Carafate for years.

What are Carafate's nasty side effects? It inhibits pepsin activity, which is crucial for the assimilation of proteins. But more important, Carafate contains aluminum, the heavy metal capable of permanently damaging the brain. In folks with less than perfect kidney function, the aluminum also displaces precious minerals in bones, leading to softening (osteomalacia) and spontaneous fractures. Further side effects include constipation, diarrhea, nausea, vomiting, gas, dry mouth, indigestion, and others. Know as well that Carafate interferes with the absorption of other drugs taken for the gut.

After reading about the side effects of these prescription drugs (see Table 2) you might be tempted to stick with nonprescription, or over-the-counter (OTC) drugs, but remember many of them only became nonprescription after their patents expired. Imodium (loperamide) is now available over the counter for diarrhea, but it's a synthetic morphine cousin so it can be addicting. Laxative abuse can occur with Metamucil, Colace, and other fiber stool softeners, while the stimulant laxatives like Dulcolax and Senokot have the potential of making you dependent on them. All in all, taking such drugs allows folks to avoid consuming real fiber in food, thereby depriving them of additional healing factors like inositol (phytic acid), shown by Dr. Shamsuddin, in his recent book *IP_6*, and by others not only to prevent, but to heal cancers.

Table 2. Side Effects and Actions of the Leading Prescription Drugs for the Gut

Brand name (and generic)	Actions	Side effects (some)
Prilosec (omeprazole) Prevacid (lansoprazole)	Proton-pump inhibitors that turn off acid secretion from stomach cells	Diarrhea, abdominal pain, nausea and vomiting, heartburn, tumors, liver death, pancreatitis, headache, back pain, serious vitamin and mineral deficiencies, anemia, infection
Propulsid (cisapride) Reglan (metoclopromide)	Hurries gastric emptying by stimulating nerve-to-gut muscle contractions	Potentially fatal ventricular tachycardia (makes the main chamber of the heart beat so abnormally that death frequently results), ventricular fibrillation (makes the other chamber beat dangerously fast, which can cause stroke), headache, diarrhea, abdominal pain, joint aches, nausea, constipation
Cytotec (misoprostol)	Cytoprotective in that it also inhibits stomach acid formation; in animals but not humans, it has been found to increase bicarbonate and mucus production	Diarrhea, abdominal pain, abortion, menstrual irregularities, nausea, vomiting, gas, headache, heartburn, constipation, depression, impotence, body aches, chest pain, arrythmia, swelling high blood pressure, blood clots, bowel bleeding, liver malfunction, deafness
Arthrotec (diclofenac and misoprostol)	A mild pain reliever (NSAID) combined with Cytotec, it's cytoprotective	
Carafate (sucralfate)	Coats stomach ulcer	Turns off pepsin needed to digest proteins; contains aluminum, the presence of which can lead to Alzheimer's, bone loss and spontaneous fractures; diarrhea, nausea; vomiting; dry mouth

Table 2. Side Effects and Actions of the Leading Prescription Drugs for the Gut (*cont.*)

Brand name (and generic)	Actions	Side effects (some)
Tagamet (cimetidine) Zantac (ranitidine) Pepcid (famotidine) Axid (nizatidine) Mylanta AR (cimetidine)	H2–blockers, turn off stomach acid. Yes, these are also available without a prescription, but the prescribed dose is higher.	Impede body detoxification thereby magnifying the side effects of other drugs and the toxic effects of environmental chemicals, arrhythmias, hypertension, gynecomastia (breast enlargement in men), headaches, liver malfunction,hair loss, anemia, infection, arthritis,and blockage of nerve conduction in the heart.

Now Let's Find the Cause before the Sick Get Any Sicker, Quicker

Yes, the traditional medical model of masking symptoms is not such a good idea after all for a number of reasons:

1. It does nothing to identify the underlying cause, so that you may need the treatment indefinitely.
2. By not finding the cause, the problem can only get worse.
3. Drugs that mask symptoms have a litany of side effects that can occur at any time, and there is no guarantee they will disappear when you stop taking the drug.
4. Such drugs interfere with proper metabolism of every other drug you take, prescription or not.
5. And worse, such drugs interfere with your body's ability to thoroughly detoxify the more than 500 potentially carcinogenic chemicals we come into contact with every day, just in our home environments alone.

The bottom line is that the gut houses over half of the body's immune system and detoxification system. These two systems govern our health. Their integrity determines every symptom and disease you get, right up to cancer. The fact is that all gut drugs make the gut malfunction. And if the gut isn't healthy, you have very little chance of healing any other condition you may have. This is a major hidden reason why many people are sick and don't get better.

The Dangers of Drugs Fall on Deaf Ears

Even as we overuse drugs and despite overwhelming evidence of the dangers they pose, physicians still seem blinded by the wonders of pharmacy. One study (Darchy), for example, showed that over one in ten admissions to hospital intensive care units (ICUs) was due to an iatrogenic or physician-caused problem, with over 40 percent the result of drug reactions, and with a 13 percent mortality rate. Now these cases included only those admitted to the ICU and recognized by a drug-oriented medical system as being iatrogenic. Cases not included in the study involve the many more patients who had general hospital admission, or no hospital admission, or who died.

In another important study, Lazarou found that drug reactions were the third cause of death in the United States, preceded by arteriosclerosis (heart attacks and strokes) and cancer. Again, the cases only reported folks who had died in the hospital under the best supervised care in the world. Not counted were all the reactions and deaths due to drugs outside the hospital, or deaths whose true cause went unrecognized. This overwhelming statistic, which should have grabbed everyone's attention when it was published in the *Journal of the American Medical Association,* didn't even rate two seconds of CNN time.

Is it any wonder that, as Eisenberg showed in another study, over one in three folks turn to at least one unconventioanal medical treatment per year? They must be sensing that drugs are not the answer to health.

Most Drugs Thwart Natural Function

The acid secretions from its cells cause the stomach to be highly acidic. This highly acidic pH has a dual function: to kill bugs that enter the mouth and to continue the digestion of food which begins in the mouth. All drugs currently used for stomach problems are anti-, or against, the natural mechanism of function, including anti-acids, or, as we know them, antacids. Years before Tagamet- and Prilosec-type drugs came on the scene, the mainstay was anticholinergic prescriptions, like Donnatal and Bentyl. They, too, were fraught with side effects, especially dry mouth, the inability to urinate, exhaustion, and psychosis.

Every drug is a blocker or an inhibitor; they all turn off normal function. The net effect on the body is negative, although it falsely makes you feel better because your symptoms are temporarily relieved. Drug-oriented medicine is not concerned with finding the cause, but with keeping you dependent on drugs that do next to nothing to cure your problem permanently while precipitating an avalanche of symptoms that only seem unrelated.

Since you are much too smart for that scheme, I guess you're left with the only rational thing to do—*find the cause*.

COMMON OTC MEDICATIONS

Just because a drug can be found on the pharmacy shelf does not mean it is safe.

Listed below are some of the more common over-the-counter gastrointestinal medications, and some of their actions and side effects (Arky, 1998).

ANTACIDS

Antacids: All antacids sop up acid, which inactivates the acid needed for digestion and nutrient absorption. Avoid those with aluminum. If you must take antacids, choose those containing magnesium or calcium.

Antacids with aluminum

Maalox	Amphogel
Di-Gel	Gaviscon
Mylanta	

Antacids with calcium, no aluminum

Tums	Alka-Mints
Titralac	Alka-Seltzer Antacid
Children's Mylanta	Rolaids

Antacids with magnesium, no aluminum

Rolaids
Phillips' Milk of Magnesia

ANTI-DIARRHEAL AGENTS

Anti-diarrheal agents: Work by slowing motility of bowel, thereby turning off nature's mechanism for getting rid of harmful bugs. Many contain aluminum, which should be avoided because it promotes Alzheimer's disease.

Anti-diarrheal with aluminum

Donnagel
Kaopectate
Pepto-Bismol

Anti-diarrheal without aluminum (potentially addicting)

Imodium

ANTI-VOMITING AGENTS

Anti-vomiting: Many are plain antihistamines which cause drowsiness. They all turn off another of nature's mechanisms to quickly get rid of harmful bugs.

Anti-vomiting agents

Dramamine	Emetrol
Bonine	Pepto-Bismol

LAXATIVES

Laxatives: The bulk-producing laxatives add fiber, which would be better obtained from real food (fruits, vegetables, and whole grains) that also contain nutrients. The more effective, but less desirable laxatives, also stimulate colon motility; the bowel can become dependent on them.

Laxatives for bulk

Metamucil	Fibercon
Perdiem	Citrucel
Konsyl	

Laxatives that also stimulate the bowel

Correctol	Dulcolax
Ex-Lax	Nature's Remedy
Senokot	Benadryl

H2-BLOCKERS

H2-Blockers: Turn off acid secretion from the cell, which impairs digestion as well as nutrient absorption and the natural antibacterial action of stomach acid. Worst of all, H2-blockers impair the detoxification pathways so that toxic side effects of drugs and environmental chemicals are magnified.

H2-Blockers

Axid	Zantac
Tagamet	Mylanta Acid Reducer
Pepcid	

CHAPTER 2

You Are What You Ate

Pain: The Body's Main Communication Mode

When you awaken at 2 A.M. after a night of overindulgence with agonizing chest and belly pain, the cause is no secret. But when, over a period of several weeks, an insidious burning slowly begins to build in your chest or in the pit of your stomach, the cause isn't so obvious.

Whenever a part of our anatomy is not happy, it reacts by sending special cells to the area to get rid of whatever has invaded or is trying to damage the resident cells. If something has been poured into the stomach that starts to burn up the lining, then the body's defense system calls out forces to protect it.

Protection in the body comes in the form of inflammation. Just as a sliver can promote a nasty inflammatory reaction in your finger, so can the wrong type of food in your stomach trigger a never-ending cascade of inflammation. As the protective inflammatory cells attempt to gobble up foreign invaders, infection, allergens, chemical additives, and any attacker causing trouble, they recruit all sorts of cells to the area, some of which cause the chemistry of pain. Inflamed tissues hurt for a reason. It is nature's way of enlisting your brain to help in solving the problem.

Simply put, pain alerts you to the fact that you are doing something wrong. Should you figure out what you did to cause the inflammation and correct it, you would probably not need to run to the drugstore or to visit your doctor. Just as the pain from touching a hot fire makes you jerk your hand away before you burn it off, the gut sends its own pain messages to tell you that you are feeding it the wrong thing. The body's role in producing pain and infmallation is merely to protect it temporarily, while you find out why you ache. Traditional medicine, however, has opted for the quick fix via drugs, making you believe your problem has been solved and that you can get on with your life without dealing with the cause of your symtoms.

Inflammation, the result of your immune cells swarming into an area to protect it, is actually labeled "-itis" in medicine. Hence an inflamed appendix ready to burst is called appendicitis, a stomach abused by the wrong foods is called gastritis, and an esophagus irritated from backflow from an overloaded stomach is called esophagitis. Since these organs lie in the vicinity of the heart, you can see why this kind of pain can be confused with heart disease or a heart condition. Therefore, in this instance at least, if at any time you are in doubt, don't wait to check it out. You can always go to an emergency room and get a cardiogram (EKG) to resolve your fears. Remember: When in doubt, check it out!

Let's look now at some of the most common causes of gastritis, or heartburn. In doing so, I'll rely on the old 80/20 rule; that is, if you examine the causes of gastritis in one hundred people, 80 percent of such causes will accord with what I give here. Most folks simply do not need a knock-down-drag-out workup. After thirty years in practice, I can safely predict that eight out of ten folks will discover what causes their ailments and how to cure them within these pages.

Cutting Out the C-R-A-P (Cigarettes, Coffee, Refined Sugars, Alcohol, Aspirin, Pop, and Processed Foods)

If you take the last hundred people with the burning, gnawing, nauseating pain of heartburn, or gastritis, a vast majority can heal themselves in less than two weeks by merely eliminating unnatural, difficult-to-digest "junk" foods that trigger the stomach to produce more acid as it struggles to digest them. Our stomachs already support the most acidic environment in the body. But it, too, has a limit as to how much it can tolerate. Too much acid, just like the chemicals of processed foods, will irritate the stomach lining, triggering a burning, inflammatory reaction.

Coffee, soda, and alcohol are our top liquid culprits. Just as you would wince from the thought of putting alcohol on an open, inflamed cut, the stomach doesn't fare any better, especially once it's inflamed. Anyone with symptoms who continues to drink coffee, soda, or alcohol may postpone healing indefinitely. Other liquid culprits are orange and other citrus juices. Drinking these on an empty morning stomach, without eating can launch an insult that the stomach will remind you of all day.

In addition, aspirin and other pain medications not only cause serious gastrointestinal (GI) burning, nausea, diarrhea, cramps, gas, and bloating, but also bleeding. Assuredly you do not want to discontinue any prescribed medications without consulting with your doctor first. But for aspirin and other related over-the-counter pain medications, like Motrin, Aleve, Advil, or Nuprin that you self-prescribe, you should certainly see if discontinuing them provides the simple solution to your tummy troubles.

Getting Over a Coffee Addiction

If asked to free associate with caffeine, you might think "coffee, quick pick-me-up, stay awake, stay alert, jitters, insomnia, addiction, heart palpitations." But would you think chronic gastritis and depression? Just remember, what goes up must come down. Just as alcohol can bring you up for a while, prolonged drinking can do the opposite. Coffee addicts, for example, are readily identified by their need for coffee at specific times, like first thing in the morning to jump-start them or at 4 P.M. to avoid a migraine or depressive slump. But the depression and migraine are merely withdrawl symptoms from the drug, caffeine. Meanwhile all this extra acidity can tear up your stomach. Nor do you need coffee to get stomach irritation from caffeine, which actually signals the stomach to make more acid! The most common sources of caffeine are listed in Table 3.

When caffeine addicts consume coffee or diet soft drinks that contain caffeine, it often exerts a calming, relaxing effect on them, since it stops caffeine withdrawal symptoms. It may even help them to sleep better, since

Table 3. Common Sources of Caffeine

Product	Serving Size	Caffeine Content
Coffee, instant	1 cup	106 mg
Coffee, percolated	1 cup	118 mg
Coffee, drip	1 cup	179 mg
Coffee, decaffeinated	1 cup	2 mg
Tea, black	1 cup	50 mg
Cola drink, regular	12 oz	60 mg
Cola drink, diet	12 oz	60 mg
Chocolate	1 oz	20 mg
Chocolate milk (cocoa)	1 cup	up to 40 mg
Anacin, Bromo Seltzer-O	1 pill	32 mg
Excedrin	1 pill	00 mg
NoDoz	1 pill	100 mg

otherwise they might go through withdrawal during the night and not be able to sleep as a result. Even though caffeine is a central nervous system stimulant, it can temporarily calm those who are addicted.

In this light, mood and energy swings are typical features of caffeine users. For example, you might have plenty of energy and be in a great mood with a general sense of well-being for a few hours after ingesting caffeine. A few hours later though, you might feel tired, depressed, and irritable. What do you do? Head for more caffeine. The result? Your good feelings return, but only to be followed by another drop in energy and a creeping depression later on. Caffeine addiction is very similar to alcohol addiction—and both tear up the stomach lining.

The only way to identify symptoms caused by an addictive substance like caffeine is to stop ingesting it long enough to get over withdrawal symptoms, and then evaluate what improves. Symptoms that have bothered you for years may disappear completely—almost certainly a sign of addiction. Whenever you find that you must have something, it generally has control over you. If you can drink caffeine every four days with no problem, merely enjoying it, then you are not hooked.

In fact, an easy test of any food addiction is to stop ingesting the particular food for four to eight days. Then eat it again, measuring your pulse before, directly after ingestion, and every ten minutes thereafter for an hour while sitting. If you consistently get a rise in pulse of ten beats per minute or more, or any other symptom, this may be an indication that your body is not happy with your food choice. And if the food in question does not produce gastric symptoms once you have healed the gut, ingesting it on a rotated basis, say once every four days, is far healthier for the body than ingesting it every day. Ingesting the food once every four days will also lessen any potential for your becomming addicted to it again.

Since dilution is the solution to pollution, drinking four to eight quarts of water a day can hasten getting over any kind of food or beverage withdrawl. Water also dilutes the acids bathing an inflamed stomach lining so that it can heal faster. The best thirst solution is chemically free noncarbonated spring water from a known good source. It should be noncarbonated, because carbonation produces an acidic reaction which also irritates the stomach. In addition, the body steals calcium from bones to neutralize or buffer the acidity that comes from carbonation. Such bodily theft of its own calcium supplies in bones can lead to osteoporosis. You should also choose glass-bottled water, since the phthalates in plastics leach into the water, which gives your body additional carcinogens to detoxify. Recent studies have shown that some of the chemicals in plastics, especially the estrogen mimics, contribute to our epidemic of breast cancer (White).

How about carrying your glass bottle of water, taken from your home water filter, to work with a lemon? You can cut fresh lemon slices throughout the day to add to the water, alkalinizing your system which also makes for clearer thinking. Often the tremendous thirst that folks sometimes experience stems from what they eat, especially if they eat salty processed foods instead of fruits, vegetables, and whole grains, which can be as much as 90 percent water. That is why we see so many folks with drinks in their hands.

In terms of water filters, none are perfect but some are better than others. Reverse osmosis (RO) and distillation are the purest. But RO wastes four to eight gallons for every one gallon produced, and distillation, while removing minerals, has limited capacity. The less expensive faucet filters miss removing some of the chemicals commonly found in the water supply. What to do?—chose what best fits your pocketbook, the area you live in, and your needs.

All home water filters are probably better than water bottled in plastic containers, which leach estrogenlike carcinogens into the water, depending on the duration and intensity of heat they were exposed to during transportation, the newness or lack of outgasing of the containers before they were filled, and more (White, Jobling). At the very least, by using home-filtered water you will know the source of the water you drink. In Chapter 7 you will also learn how to test your water for unwanted chemicals.

Meanwhile, caffeine is clearly an example of one of many food constituents (not unlike sugar and fake sugars, MSG and other additives, dyes and preservatives) that can have a profound effect not only on the stomach but on brain chemistry. And let's not forget another culprit that isn't even a food. Every time you put a cigarette in your mouth, your stomach thinks it is going to be getting food. So it gears up in anticipation and begins to secrete extra acid, which can keep gastritis smoldering.

What Drives You to Eat the Wrong Foods?

As you travel to work, look around you at the folks carrying soda cans. When did we suddenly become a nation in need of a constant infusion of sugar, dyes, and artificial ingredients? Part of the addiction stems from hypoglycemia, commonly called low blood sugar.

If you must have something in your mouth every hour or so, you may have defective sugar and energy metabolism from deficiencies of vanadium, manganese, chromium, L-carnitine, thioctic acid, or magnesium. In some folks the pancreas is an allergic target organ. Just as the nose runs when exposed to airborne mold, the pancreas secretes when triggered to do so. Only its secretion is not mucus, but insulin, causing hypoglycemia instead of a runny nose. Symptoms then can vary from dizziness, weakness, sweats, headache, or jitteriness to unexplained mood swings and sudden unprovoked personality changes. People can kill for sugar when that insulin rush drives their glucose level down.

Food allergy is another common trigger causing the pancreas to malfunction. In fact, an allergy to milk (lactose intolerance) has contributed to some cases of juvenile diabetes. Other triggers for hunger and thirst, which can also cause the pancreas to secrete too much insulin and produce hypoglycemia, include anxiety, alcoholism, fatty acid or mineral deficiencies, environmental chemicals, a gut full of yeast, or diabetes itself. At times, of course, an individual just may not drink enough water to satiate his or her thirst as compensation for ingesting so many processed foods and chemicals, and to dilute gastric acid.

Vanadium to the Sugar Craver's Rescue

Do you have sugar cravings? Do you constantly fill your stomach with processed foods to satisfy your sugar cravings? Do you exercise but the pounds linger? Do you also have any arteriosclerosis in the form of heart disease, high blood pressure, congestive heart failure, or heart arrhythmia? Or do you have diabetes, hypoglycemia, or chronic fatigue? If so, you probably do not get 200 to 400 micrograms of vanadium a day. Yet it could be a life saver and help you reduce weight, blood pressure, insulin requirements, and rev up your energy, along with helping cure the cravings for junk food that can irritate your stomach.

Much evidence shows that vanadium is a unique mineral that mimics insulin in the body (Bhanoit, Verma). So if you are an insulin-dependent diabetic and wish to take vanadium as a dietary supplement, proceed with caution. By satisfying your daily requirement for vanadium, you may require as much as two-thirds less insulin than you are used to. If, however, while on vanadium supplements you start to get depressed, then back off or stop taking them completely. Trying to correct a deficiency too quickly can lower lithium and other delicate mineral balances that affect brain chemistry. Vanadium also works better in concert with other nutrients known to decrease cravings for sweets, like chromium, L-carnitine, and manganese.

For safe slow correction of your sugar cravings, I would suggest 100 to 250 micrograms of supplemental vanadium every or every other day over one to six months. This regimen is recommended for people who have not previously measured their vanadium levels, and who do not have kidney disease or an otherwise delicate balance. Vanadian Krebs (N.E.E.D.S.) is an excellent, inexpensive, organic form containing 250 micrograms attached to citrate, malate, fumarate, glutarate, and succinate molecules. Vanadium Krebs could also be combined with 200 micrograms of Chromium Cruciferate (Ecologic Formulas), L-Carnitine 500 milligrams (Pure Encapsulations or Jarrow), Manganese Picolinate 20 mg (Thorne), glycine (Pain & Stress) and one Multiplex-1 without Iron (Tyler) for starters to begin to correct some of the leading deficiencies that trigger sugar cravings.

The Chromium Cycle of Sugar Cravings

Another way the body relentlessly causes cravings involves what I call the chromium cycle. Chromium is a trace mineral needed by the body to control hypoglycemia (low blood sugar) as well as diabetes (high blood sugar). When animals lack a mineral, they forage for the missing element, gnawing on the bark of some tree or grazing in a new pasture. But humans, having sacrificed their instincts on the altar of fast foods, usually forage in the freezer for Häagen-Dazs and the like.

Delicious as Häagen-Dazs may be, eating it does not fix the problem but only exacerbates it. Unfortunately, the more sugar an individual eats, the more chromium he or she loses in the urine, so the vicious cycle of cravings, even leading to obesity, is launched (Kozlovsky, AS, et al). That is one reason why you never see obese animals in the wild, and certainly never see them sucking down sodas or Mylanta. Animals instinctively fix what is broken.

The Hyperacidity Myth

A trip through any shopping mall food court shows the dazzling array of plastic processed foods available. Are our stomachs meant for such a vast array of foods combined with overindulgence? I should say not. We often eat as though there were no tomorrow. But when a large bolus of food arrives in the stomach, if it contains chemical preservatives foreign to the body, if there has been insufficient chewing providing predigestion, or if there are insufficient enzymes to process the mass, it can just sit there, with fermentation or bacterial action the result. As the gases rise, they get trapped in and distend the esophagus, mimicking chest pain. The tension and pull of the overloaded stomach stresses the gastroesophageal valve to the point that it's pulled open. This overstretched valve not only allows gases up into the esophagus, but allows a back surge or reflux of stomach acid, perhaps with some stomach contents, into the esophagus as well.

The stomach is lined with acid-secreting cells, but the esophagus is not. In fact, the esophagus is very sensitive to acid. So when gases, stomach acid, or partially digested food slide back up into the esophagus, even a tiny amount is perceived by the delicate esophageal tissues as way too much.

With a burning sensation now localized to the esophagus, we can all too easily interpret it as a stomach upset, a stomach with too much acid, when the reality is quite different. Often there is too little acid in the stomach to complete the oversized job of digestion. Taking an antacid or other medications to inhibit the secretion of stomach acid then makes no sense; except for the companies that produce the pill or liquid.

Recently, Tums has been touted not only as a good antacid, but as a source of calcium. But think about it. Tums is calcium carbonate, or chalk. It works to quell an inflamed stomach by sopping up acid. Nonetheless, the body needs acid to help it absorb calcium. So how much calcium can be absorbed? Not much at all. Furthermore, for years medical studies have shown that when you use milk or antacids to sop up acid, the stomach "rebounds" or compensates by sending out extra acid next time.

First Steps for Improving Your Digestion

If you present hyperacidity symptoms to the stomach specialist, the first thing he or she will want to do is take a peek. So let's look at some of the common, simple and inexpensive things you can do long before you resort to esophagoscopy. If you would prefer not having a three-foot scope inserted down into your stomach, begin where digestion begins, in the head. Make sure mealtime is peaceful, not stressed by channel surfing, violent videos, or unpleasant conversations.

Next, chew each mouthful of food at least ten to fifty times. The number of times will depend on the condition of your teeth, the kind of food you are eating, and how sick you are. Did you know that there are folks who are so sick that they need to chew each mouthful until it is totally liquid in order to begin to heal?

Although the salivary and parotid glands are meant to initiate digestion, we seem not to understand that simple fact. In the current era, it is far too common to see folks chew two to three times and swallow. Look around you and count how many times folks chew before they swallow. Some look like they don't even chew at all. How many times do you chew before you swallow? If you are accustomed to two to five chews and bolting down your food, then try doubling the chews for a week. Then see if you can triple them. For mixing food well with saliva is the first step to digestion, and slow peaceful chewing fosters the secretion of enzymes to make sure you get the most from your food with the fewest symptoms. Appropriate chewing also allows you to listen to what others have a burning desire to tell you.

Food combining is a technique that is successfully used by some people to stop indigestion, gas, and bloating, as well as to lose weight. With this plan you merely cut back from eating many dissimilar foods at one sitting. The result is clear: You don't overtax the capability of your digestive enzymes. As with any diet program, there are all sorts of levels or degrees of restriction. Fortunately most folks do not have to be very strict, but they can benefit from the principles used by those who do in order to heal themselves.

For example, serious food combiners never eat fruit with other foods, but save it for a solo meal like breakfast, a light dinner, or a between meals snack. The idea is simple: If starches and proteins are eaten with fruits, they require lengthier digestion. As a result, the fruits, which are along for the ride but are delayed in the gut, begin to ferment, resulting in gas and bloating. If the meal includes more quickly digestible fruits that are detained in the gut because they accompany slower digesting foods like meats or potatoes, fermentation action between gut bacteria, gut yeasts, and fruits can lead to the production of gas.

As the gases distend the gut wall, they cause painful bloating, cramps, uncomfortable fullness, and indigestion. They can also turn toxic to the tissues and nerves, causing an inflammatory reaction that impairs the normal, peristaltic wave action initiated by gut nerves to propel food along. This adds constipation to the bloating and cramps.

Food-combining rules can be intensely limiting and there is little scientific evidence that various types of foods inhibit the secretion of certain digestive enzymes, which as you learned in the preceding chapter are so plentiful. If food combining is for you, however, then try it. In addition, many recommendations by those who follow food combining, as the soaking and/or sprouting of grains, legumes (beans), seeds, and nuts definitely improves an individual's ability to chew them, digest them, and absorb their live enzymes and nutrients.

For novices at food combining, why not start with mono meals, even if just as a trial. Eat only one food per meal to see how the body tolerates it. Then you can slowly add two types of foods that you can tolerate to see how your body responds to specific food combinations. This is the best test of your individual chemistry and digestive abilities at this point in time. For after you become well and know how and why you did so, you will probably not need to be concerned about what foods to eat when.

When you do a mono meal trial, make sure the food is wholesome. Breakfast could be your fruit meal: papaya, watermelon, or bananas. But if you are unsatisfied because you must have protein, add some eggs or lox (smoked salmon). For lunch, why not try sweet potatoes, squash, or a big salad of grated vegetables. Again, however, if you are a closet carnivore and must have some high-quality protein, then you may have to break the food-combining rules a bit and include a can of Alaskan salmon, for example, in your salad. For dinner, broccoli, brown rice, with an organic roasted free range chicken is delicious. As you increase your tolerance, you can add more foods.

Pure food is the key, which leaves out junk foods, additives, or foods ground, crushed, mashed, or otherwise mutilated by some machine. If, in your elimination diet, you rule out butter intolerance (have no butter for four days, then pile it on the next day and evaluate symptoms), then you can test your tolerance to sea salt and black pepper to improve the palatability of the vegetables you'll eat more and more often. The same goes for olive oil, lemon juice, and fresh herbs like garlic, basil, cilantro, or thyme.

The operative word here is *individuality*. As much as medicine would like us to believe that we are all the same, we are not. You must discover what foods make and keep you healthy, along with how pleasurable they can taste. For folks who find that food combining is a real help and want more definitive information, then Harvey and Marilyn Diamond's *Fit for Life* and Rita Romano's *Dining in the Raw* are for you.

Processed Foods Hide Potent Triggers of Inflammation

Besides having over 80 percent of the natural nutrients needed for healing the gut removed, processed foods like those containing bleached white flour, sugar, or hydrogenated oils can cause food allergies that inflame the gut. What processed foods do contain is just as important as what they do not contain. Let's look at a few of the hidden additives the average person eats many times a day.

Myth: There Is Safety in Low-Fat Foods

You may find it as difficult as I did to learn that our government is not protecting us from harmful food additives. For example, there is Olestra, the recently released fat substitute. Because food manufacturers plan on allowing Olestra to permeate the food system much as they did with the health-destroying hydrogenated "trans" fatty acids, you will have to be more careful than ever. As a fat substitute, Olestra will be hidden in a banquet of processed foods from cookies, breads, salad dressings, and cold cuts to cheese dishes, "health shakes," "healthy" gourmet-style instant meals, chips, bagels, and pretzels. In fact, any food that boasts being "lite," low in calories, low fat, or guilt-free is suspect.

What is the problem with Olestra? This fake fat cannot be absorbed by the body and it also inhibits the absorption of the most important cancer-preventing, fat-soluble vitamins like E, A, D, and K, as well as beta-carotene. These nutrients, crucial for maintaining our everyday health, are indispensable for healing the gut. Clearly, the introduction of Olestra into the food system is guaranteed to increase our already-unrecognized epidemic of nutrient deficiencies and undiagnosable diseases. One study even shows Olestra decreasing an individual's vitamin D level by 19 percent in just six weeks of eating cookies laced with it daily (Jones). This is not what the doctor ordered for people who live in cloudy northern cities (where lack of sunlight can cause a vitamin D deficiency) or for a nation that is already plagued with osteoporosis and half of whose citizens over fifty-five have lost their teeth.

In terms of understanding how Olestra, and other like substances, are approved as food additives, I reviewed the scientific studies that were done on it, studies that enabled the manufacturer, Procter & Gamble, to get Food and Drug Administration (FDA) approval. In one study the manufacturer wanted to prove that Olestra was nontoxic and did not cause cancer (Miller). But because it is known that Olestra inhibits the absorption of fat-soluble vitamins that every animal, including humans, must have to prevent cancer, the mice used in the Olestra trial also had extra vitamins A, D, E, and K added to their diets. The control mice did not. Now this is unheard of in real science. You *never* give the test group a distinct advantage over the control group. In fact, this advantage negates the entire reason for the control group. You may not be surprised to find out that the study for Olestra's FDA approval was done by Procter & Gamble, the very people who make Olestra. That's like asking the fox to guard the hen house.

The conclusion reached at the end of this one-year study surprised no one. Olestra, it was said, caused no problem. Again, the animals were supplemented with the same vitamins that Olestra lowers. Unfortunately the American public who eats Olestra may not be supplemented like the lucky mice. Some manufacturers claim that they will add vitamin E to the Olestra, so there is nothing to worry about. But when vitamin E is added back to foods, the dose of less than 30 I.U. is ridiculously low. The recommended daily allowance (RDA) for vitamin E now stands at 400 to 800 I.U. (international units), the amount needed to dramatically cut the risk of heart disease and cancer. Also, the form of vitamin E chosen by food manufacturers is the cheap, synthetic type, commonly used by the drug industry in grocery store nutrients of inferior dose and quality. The body is unable to use or to metabolize over half of the synthetic form, since its molecular structure is so foreign to our chemistry. Compared with natural sources of high-quality, health store vitamin E, there is no contest.

Let's look at another "safety" study on Olestra (Lafrancon). In this study, researchers used dogs instead of mice. But again, they supplemented the dog diets with extra vitamins A and E. The conclusion replicated that of the previous study. Olestra is not toxic. But for a human, who may not get these added nutrients, after a few months of eating chips or cookies laced with Olestra, there may be an insidious onset of vitamin E deficiency. Since vit-

amin E protects cell membranes against chemical assault, the victim will
be much more vulnerable to developing gut toxicity to anything in his or
her diet, such as carcinogenic pesticides and additives.

Again, it was Procter & Gamble that conducted this "safety" study. If I
had not read the actual reports, I frankly do not think I would have believed
it. But you can see for yourselves the incredible "science" that makes up
the "safe" studies for food additives. And when I heard the announcement
on TV "that the FDA had approved Olestra as a new fat substitute," I was
appalled. The TV announcement also made the claim that studies in mice
and dogs showed Olestra to be perfectly safe. With Olestra, the announcement continued, "you can have delicious desserts with half the calories and
not have to worry. And you can party with guilt-free chips and pretzels
each night."

Food products containing Olestra will be termed healthy, fat-free, or low
in fat. Yet such food products are usually also accompanied by fake sugars,
hydrogenated vegetable oils containing trans fatty acids known to advance
premature arteriosclerosis and heart attacks, not to mention a plethora of
assorted additives, preservatives, pesticides, dyes, and more.

Harvard scientists have also shown that just fifteen to twenty Olestra
potato chips a day can drop your beta-carotene level by a monstrous 60 percent (Blundell). Beta-carotene, of course, is a major nutrient for cancer and
arteriosclerosis prevention, as well as for healing the gut. In fact, Harvard
scientists have caused cancers to revert to normal cells with high doses of
beta-carotene.

So now we know. Olestra, this "wonderful new fat substitute," stifles nutrient absorption for vitamins A, D, E, K, beta-carotene, and the tocotrienols, and along with the already nutrient-poor quality of the food
product and its other hidden additives makes for very unhealthy eating. As
we know, most potato chips are prepared with trans fatty acids which directly damage cell membranes. The guilt-free pretzel is made from
bleached, processed white flour that has been purposely stripped of its healing and protective vitamins E and B_6, magnesium, molybdenum, and manganese—all so that it can be kept in the pantry indefinitely without going
bad. You can think of this another way. If most of the natural "goodness"
that bugs need to sustain themselves is removed from food products, what
self-respecting bacteria or fungus is going to invade that food? They know
better. They won't eat that junk—it will slowly kill them.

I hope the scenario of a slow deterioration in health that I've suggested is
enough to convince you that Olestra, among other food additives, *is not
good for you.* If you believe otherwise, be careful, for Olestra's major side
effect is loose stools or diarrhea. The addition of Olestra to our food supply

is one more way to silently erode the health of consumers while making sure they have enough ailments to support the drug industry.

Diarrhea, gastritis, or any gut symptom can be the result of any of the many, in fact, hundreds, of food additives used today. Just remember: Nature does not have to advertise or brag. Whole foods have the nutritional content you need to be healthy, and they do not require a label. If there is a label, you are probably in the wrong territory. Food marketed as guilt-free fare is always suspicious. Any time claims are made that a food product is low in fat or has been fortified with nutrients, think twice about ingesting it until you know what it is, where it came from, and what it does.

Olestra does not always go by the same name. Some of its aliases include sucrose octaoleate, sucrose polyester, and olean. Other aliases will certainly come along as well. In the meantime, it's just better and healthier to avoid low-fat, low-calorie, or guilt-free foods until you investigate them for safety. Most likely they will contain the new fat substitutes. You are always safer with a whole, unadulterated food that does not require a label. Then, too, you cannot live without fat, and I mean the good, essential fats from whole grains, vegetables, seeds, nuts, and animals. Good fats are cold pressed, protected from heat and light, and have not been processed into trans fatty acids (like margarine) or hydrogenated oils. Good fats are a necessary part of the backbone of life and for any healing of the gut.

Monosodium Glutamate (MSG): Toxin at the Table

An even more common food additive, monosodium glutamate (MSG), can also cause diarrhea, nausea, vomiting, or mimic the kind of any gastric or irritable bowel symptoms. Yet rare is the gastroenterologist who would take you off all processed foods for a trial to determine if MSG is the cause of your gut symptoms.

As we feed the world, food needs to last longer for shipping and storage. And as foods lose their natural tastes through processing, they must be substituted with artificial tastes. MSG may sound pretty innocuous, but as board-certified and practicing neurosurgeon Russell Blaylock, explained, it can reproduce just about every symptom there is.

Belonging to a category of food additives that are called excitotoxins, MSG revs up brain amino acids that make one feel "up," stimulated, or slightly excited, leading to possible addictive eating patterns and subsequent obesity. Dr. Blaylock stumbled onto this research when he found that his very own children were so hooked on a particular Chef Boyardee spaghetti sauce with pasta alphabets that they craved it for every meal. He found that it was the MSG that provoked the craving reaction in his children.

As his research led him deeper into the chemistry of MSG, Dr. Blaylock was startled to find that, through hyperstimulation, MSG actually wears out the nerves: MSG and related food additives can destroy the nerve cells, specifically in the inner layers of the retina, or back of the eyeball, and in the hypothalamic area of the brain that controls, among other things, the glandular functions in the body. Dr. Blaylock also found that as little as a single dose of MSG can trigger nerve deterioration.

Since there are no tests for MSG addiction or damage, complaints are often chalked up to hypochondriasis. As symptoms increase, diagnoses such as irritable bowel syndrome, nervous colitis, spastic colon, hypoglycemia, hyperactivity, learning disability, depression, unexplained mood swings, confusion, seizures, migraines, strokes, and dementia are made.

By the time the nerve destruction has reached diagnosable proportions, even more serious labels such as Alzheimer's, amyotrophic lateral sclerosis (ALS), stroke, seizures, migraine, Huntington's chorea, or Parkinson's disease come forth. These suggest that not much can be offered except more prescription drugs to quell some of the presenting symptoms. Another chemical on board, however, is the last thing the struggling detoxification systems of these people need.

MSG is being added to more and more of the foods we eat, causing symptoms that occur immediately or insidiously. It may accumulate silently for years before the destruction of brain cells occurs. Fortunately, not everyone is vulnerable, but there is no test that can reveal who is.

Because MSG can be cloaked in such benign-sounding terms as caseinate, natural flavoring, autolyzed yeast, spices, hydrolyzed soy protein, or hydrolyzed vegetable protein, it is rarely suspected as a culprit. In addition, overt symptoms may be delayed in appearance by as many as two days after ingestion, making the correct diagnosis even more unlikely.

Food Additives: What You See Isn't Necessarily What You Get

Here is a primary way that MSG can slip into foods without appearing on the label. The last person on the train of manufacturers who had a role in making a particular processed food may buy, for example, some hydrolyzed vegetable protein. You have seen this on lots of labels. It is made from left over "junk" vegetables that are unfit for sale or from peelings that would otherwise be discarded. They are boiled (hydrolyzed) in a vat of acid, then neutralized with caustic soda.

Don't believe everything you read. Unfortunately it is not easy to avoid MSG, because U.S. government FDA product laws appear to favor the manufacturer over the consumer here as well. FDA product laws allow manufacturers to specifically state "No MSG," and "No added MSG," and "No MSG added" (section 403, a,1 of the Federal Food and Drug, and Cosmetic Act), on packages even when those products still contain MSG. Through the successful lobbying clout of major food brand giants, a clairvoyant government advisory panel has decided that they know exactly how much of any particular food product you would ingest in any one day. If their presumed knowledge of your food habits, allergies, individual biochemistry, environmental overload, and genetic predisposition is correct, then the amount of MSG, for example, in a particular food labeled "No MSG" should not bother you. What happens if you should get hooked on a food and eat more of it than they imagined does not seem to be a concern.

The result, a brown sludge that collects on the top, is scraped off and allowed to dry. The resulting powder, which contains glutamate, is then sold for use in processed foods. But since the last person to add it is not actually adding MSG, but protein hydrolysate, he or she does not have to mention that it contains glutamate, even though assay confirms its significant presence.

Soups, sauces, gravies, and bouillon cubes, as well as most diet foods, almost always contain it, because foods low in fat are even more bland without taste enhancers like MSG. Everything from canned tuna to baby food can contain it—and the immature developing brain is one of the last places we want it. But people, including infants, become addicted to processed foods that contain MSG as a taste enhancer, making them vulnerable to the side effects of numerous gut symptoms.

Of course, there are occasions when a super-sensitivity to MSG (as in Chinese restaurant syndrome) can disappear because the way the body detoxifies it has been repaired. The most common nutrients that have accomplished this (bear in mind everyone has a different defect) have been molybdenum, magnesium, and vitamins B_{12} and B_6.

From Table 4, you can appreciate that the only way to avoid MSG is to eat whole, unprocessed foods, and nothing in a box, bag, jar, or wrapper that has foreign or chemical-sounding names that you cannot readily define. Recall these three important points as well:

1. Addictive additives are everywhere in the food supply; in fact, there are thousands of such additives.
2. Additives are cloaked in different chemical names, while creative interpretation of food-manufacturing laws makes their identification even more difficult.
3. Additives have far-reaching side effects, not the least of which is causing many different kinds of gut symptoms.

Table 4. Sources of MSG

These names mean MSG:

Glutamate	Textured protein
Monosodium glutamate	Hydrolyzed protein (any protein that is
Monopotassium glutamate	hydrolyzed)
Glutamic acid	Yeast extract
Calcium caseinate	Yeast food
Sodium caseinate	Autolyzed yeast
Gelatin	Yeast nutrient

These often contain MSG or create MSG during processing:

Malt extract	Whey protein concentrate	Seasonings (the word "seasonings")
Malt flavoring	Pectin	Soy sauce
Barley malt	Protease enzymes	Soy protein
extract	Enzymes	Soy protein isolate
Bouillon cubes	Protease	anything protein-fortified
Stock	Flavor(s) and Flavoring(s)	anything enzyme modified
Broth	Natural flavor(s)	anything ultrapasteurized
Carrageenan	Natural pork flavoring	anything fermented
Maltodextrin	Natural beef flavoring	
Whey protein	Natural chicken flavoring	
Whey protein isolate		

Don't pass up an opportunity to determine whether or not MSG is causing your GI symptoms. (See Table 5.) If you do, you may just be sentencing yourself to a lifetime of needless medications that only temporarily mask symptoms.

The Not-So-Sweet NutraSweet

Eliminating fake sugar should also be one of your goals. Aspartame goes under the familiar names of Equal or NutraSweet and it is usually hidden in products labeled "contains no sugar," "lite," "low in calories," or "dietetic." Once again, the more the wrapper has to brag about, the less you are probably going to want it.

Aspartame is composed of two amino acids, phenylalanine and aspartic acid. Now phenylalanine competes with tryptophan, which lowers tryptophan levels in the brain. Since tryptophan is the primary amino acid for synthesis of one of our brain's hormones that trigger elation of mood, or a happy feeling, aspartame has contributed to depression in some individuals, as well as insomnia, headaches, dizziness, or mood swings. In fact, if it was possible to measure how much the ubiquitous appearance of aspartame packets at restaurants affects the current Prozac epidemic, the result would be interesting.

Table 5. MSG Symptoms

Cardiac
Arrhythmias
Extreme drop in blood pressure
Rapid heartbeat (tachycardia)
Angina

Circulatory
Swelling/fluid retention

Muscular
Flu-like achiness
Joint pain
Stiffness

Neurological
Depression
Dizziness, light-headedness
Loss of balance
Disorientation, mental confusion
Anxiety, panic attacks
Hyperactivity, behavioral
problems in children
Lethargy, sleepiness, insomnia
Migraine headache
Numbness or paralysis
Seizure
Sciatica
Slurred speech

Gastrointestinal
Diarrhea
Nausea/vomiting
Stomach cramps
Irritable bowel
Bloating

Respiratory
Asthma (shortness of breath)
Chest pain, tightness

Skin
Hives or rash
Mouth lesions
Temporary tightness or partial paralysis (numbness
or tingling) of the skin
Flushing
Extreme dryness of the mouth

Urological
Swelling of prostate
Nocturia (frequent nightly urination)

Visual
Blurred vision
Difficulty focusing

Source: Blaylock, RL, *Excitotoxins: The Taste That Kills,* Santa Fe, NM: Health Press, 1994. (Highly recommended.)

But there are other problems with aspartame. For example, if we do not get a surge of tryptophan after a meal, we often do not feel satisfied or satiated. Hence, many people using fake sugars for weight reduction increase rather than diminish their cravings, and actually eat more than they normally would. One study has even confirmed the rebound to increased hunger after eating aspartame-laced foods, as though the body knew it had been duped (Drenowski, Rogers). As a result, we have a generation of folks going out of their way to eat fake sugars to help them lose weight, only to find themselves eating more and gaining more weight.

If depression and cravings are not enough reason to stop using aspartame, its molecular structure should be. Aspartame's two amino acids are held together with a methanol molecule that is metabolized in the body to produce formaldehyde. This can cause headache, mood swings, brain fog, and dizziness, and it can also mimic gut symptoms. It makes more sense to use the natural herb, stevia (see next chapter for a source) which substitutes for sugar without producing calories, caries, or Candida!

Furthermore, aspartame has been closely linked to the epidemic of thyroid abnormalities like Graves' disease and thyroiditis. In cases where aspartame use accompanied Graves' disease, patients went into remission as thyroid function improved following an unplanned rest from the culprit, aspartame. When they re-introduced aspartame into their diets, however, their thyroiditis recurred (Roberts).

Yes, we are the experimental generation for all these new chemicals in our food and drink. Once you arm yourself with enough of the facts, however, it makes doing the right thing a breeze. I bet that next time you see aspartame on a food label or go to reach for the little pink or blue packets on the restaurant table, you'll think twice about the dangers hidden in a chemical that merely allows us to eat more of something that probably has little or no redeeming value to begin with. For aspartame is just one more way of getting you hooked on nutrient-depleted, additive-laced foods that cause the mimicking of gut symptoms and retard healing of the gut once you discover the cause.

What about Saccharin?

Cheaper than aspartame, saccharin leaves a bitter aftertaste. And like other fake sugars, it cannot fool the body. A rebound of increased hunger was noticed in those who had eaten food with saccharin, but there was no similar hunger when the same food was consumed without it (Blundell).

Being 300 times sweeter than sugar, saccharin gave aspartame competition until it was implicated in triggering bladder cancer. After being vindicated by subsequent studies (some of which were industry-supported or flawed in their methodology) saccharin is now making a comeback. Would I recommend it? Not a chance. As a synthetic compound derived from coal tar, taking saccharin is asking for cancer.

Don't forget this fact either: When 500 mice with breast cancer are needed for research, giving one dose of a coal tar compound to each mouse is sufficient for them to get cancer. With all the carcinogens we are exposed to every day, it simply makes no sense to ingest one intentionally. And again, of what value is a processed food that has to have saccharin added in the first place? If it's a treat, go ahead and enjoy it with real sugar. Better yet, make your own with honey, maple syrup, yinnie rice syrup, or use the herb stevia.

The Dangers of Unseen Additives: The Great Medical Mimics

"What you don't know won't hurt you." I don't know where that phrase originated, but it appears to be an appropriate slogan for food manufacturers. Each day millions of Americans devour foods loaded with chemicals whose names they don't recognize—and wouldn't have the foggiest notion of what they mean. But what is more alarming is that most of these additives are capable of creating symptoms that mimic diseases. In a society where disease usually equates a deficiency of some prescribed drug, this can initiate the downward spiral of symptom→drug→side effect, new symptom→worsening of the old symptom, and—since the cause is still not looked for—new drug→new symptom, etc.

Let's look at the onslaught. Routinely used food chemicals include coloring agents, preservatives, antioxidants, stabilizers, gelifiers, binders, thickeners, flavoring agents, taste enhancers, sweeteners, yeast and enzymes used for hydrogenation, catalysts, cooling by contact, extraction by solvents, lubrication, propulsive agents, resin ion exchangers, and unmolding agents. In an era of increasingly informed consumers, it is strange that the vast majority still eat foods that contain chemicals that they have never heard of. Then, too, what is not on the label may outrank what is, like heavy metal toxicity from aluminum cooking vats or pesticides used for storage and shipping of raw materials.

The gut was designed for absorbing nutritious food, not foreign chemicals. Once you find the causes for your symptoms, you need all the nutrients found in food but lacking in "plastic," chemicalized, processed foods to heal it. Furthermore, whole nutritious foods are needed to keep the gut healthy once it is healed.

Some additives also contain parts of foods to which an individual may have an allergy. For example, Simplesse, used in many cream-based desserts, mayonnaises, and salad dressings as a replacement for fat, has the allergenicity of its milk and egg proteins.

Just as nearly all prescribed and nonprescription medications have side effects predominating with gut symptoms, so do many chemical additives. The Chinese restaurant syndrome, caused by MSG by decreasing plasma cholinesterase, an enzyme crucial in nerve chemistry, can mimic all the side effects of pesticide poisoning. The resulting massive histamine release can also cause many symptoms, from migraine or paresthesias (numbness and tingling) to chest pain mimicking a heart attack, depression, or brain fog. Just as common a symptom here is epigastric (pit of the stomach) pain.

Tyramine, an amino acid that occurs naturally in foods, can cause mysterious and serious gut pain as well. Low doses of tyramine, for example, found in certain cheeses, can lead not only to severe stomach pain, but also to massive histamine release which causes headaches, hypertensive crisis, stroke, or death, especially in those who are genetically predisposed to such a reaction or who are on specific prescribed antidepressants. Since we live in a society where discovering the cause is rarely emphasized, but drugs are frequently prescribed to suppress symptoms, the real cause here is often missed.

Antioxidants are little different. When placed in foods (e.g., sodium nitrate in hot dogs, vanillin in cream, BHT and BHA in boxed cereals, etc.), antioxidants can cause stomach pain, specifically by inhibiting diamine oxidase—an enzyme that normally metabolizes food histamines. If they are not metabolized, food histamines back up and cause myriad symptoms, including heartburn, nausea, indigestion, pain, gas, bloating, diarrhea, or constipation. Of equal importance is the extra work that your body must do to detoxify each and every chemical it encounters. When important nutrients are used up to detoxify chemical food additives, they will not be available to help prevent environmental chemicals from causing the genetic changes that initiate cancer, promote depression, or retard healing of the gut.

Research abounds showing ways that food additives also destroy what remaining nutrients there may be in processed foods (Cort). For example, sulfur dioxide, used to preserve dried fruits, can cleave (i.e., break apart) and inactivate vitamin B_1 (thiamin) and folic acid. Thiamin is destroyed in alkaline foods such as chocolate cake, baked goods packaged in aluminum, baking powder, and tortillas. Is it any wonder that we find the vitamin B_1 deficiency that contributes to chronic fatigue so common?

The bottom line is this: Be aware, be advised, and eat as few processed foods with their lists of strange ingredients as possible. The rule of thumb here—if you do not know what an ingredient is, why eat it? Remember, if a food lists its ingredients, it means something of the natural goodness, nutritional status, or flavor has been sacrificed in lieu of prolonged shelf life. You are better off with a pure, fresh, whole fruit, vegetable, or organic food and meat.

Are You Aware of the Cereal Killer in Your Pantry?

Entire grocery store aisles are lined with them, unsuspecting shoppers carry them home to the pantries of U.S. households. Each morning millions of Americans unknowingly start their day with a cereal killer. Look at the label of your cereal box. Does it contain dead, processed, bleached, enriched, broken grains, sugars, synthetic vitamins, chemical additives, dyes, and hydrogenated trans fatty acid oils (usually soybean oil) as the majority do? Because boxed cereal plays such a steady role in most Americans' diets, it has a profound influence on accelerating disease.

Any food, for example, that contains hydrogenated oils also contains some trans fatty acids that actually hurry heart disease, cancer, and aging. In addition, they slow the healing of the gut as well as make it more vulnerable to deterioration. Fortunately, natural oils that are cold pressed, like extra virgin olive oil, do not undergo hydrogenation. But soybean, cottonseed, and other vegetable oils used in processed foods, especially cereals, are hydrogenated. Why is this bad? The process of hydrogenation exposes a once healthful oil to extremely high temperatures, which causes its molecules to twist into a very unnatural trans isomer. When you consume this unnatural trans isomer and incorporate it into your cell membranes, it will distort their functions in the most unpredictable ways. A lifetime of french fries, white breads with hydrogenated oils, margarines, salad dressings, and myriad other like foods leads to a steady but definite decline in health.

I cringe when I see huge letters on cereal boxes, bragging that the cereal is fortified with an irresistible amount of nutrients. Foods that need to be fortified, however, are foods whose processing, bleaching, and storage have previously depleted them of those same nutrients. The deception is clear. Add to this the fact the daily RDA is grossly underestimated, especially when nutrients are expressed as a percentage, and our concerns rise even more. Being made to look appealing or good for you does not mean that the cereal is a healthy food.

For as soon as a whole grain is cut or broken in any way, its nutrient value starts to deteriorate. Just imagine how dead, devitalized, and loaded with preservatives cereal must be to last in a box for months on end. Could you create any type of grain product in your own kitchen that would last in a box for as long without spoiling? Notice as well that not even grain moths or other insects are interested in it, except perhaps sugar ants.

Sugar is a multifaced culprit, with many roles to play in undermining your health. Sugar causes a rise in insulin, thereby creating hunger and cravings. This rise in insulin then causes unused sugar to be stored as fat, which contributes to obesity; in addition, this increase in insulin stimulates the liver to produce cholesterol—the real villain behind arteriosclerosis, the number one killer in the United States.

Another mechanism by which sugar contributes to arteriosclerosis is through glycosylation of proteins. Sugar hooks onto (or glycosylates) other body proteins, damaging their key roles in preventing arteriosclerosis. Sugar also robs the body of nutrients that could have been ingested in whole foods. Foods that need to glamorize themselves with sucrose to make them more appealing are notoriously low in other nutrients. Sugar-laden products often contain trans fatty acids as well, which contribute to premature deterioration of the cell membranes where hormone receptors are located. This deterioration leads to insulin resistance, which then can cause anything from poor healing of gut tissues to cravings, obesity or chronic fatigue.

If that were not reason enough to ban fake foods from your first meal of the day, there is another problem hidden in sugars. Slowly over time, many folks stop making special enzymes called disaccharidases that properly break down or metabolize sugar. This decrease in production is caused by such factors as aging, gut infections and gut medications. The result is gas bloating, indigestion, and major gut disturbance. In contrast, glucose is a monosaccharide. It is the sugar found in honey, and does not cause the digestive problems that table sugar or sucrose does, which is a disaccharide, or double sugar (breaks down to form glucose and fructose). Therefore, substituting honey can stop gut problems that regular sugar causes.

Buck-flower cereal is cheaper and infinitely more nutritious than prepackaged, store-bought cereal. Before you retire at night, put a small handful each of sunflower seeds and buckwheat groats in your bowl. Add enough spring water to cover; overnight soaking lowers phytates and promotes digestibility. By morning the cereal will be ready to eat. Merely rinse the seeds again sometime the next day—they will begin to sprout, and can still be used for cereal the next day or, you can continue to sprout them to use in salads, sandwiches, or as garnish. For the soaked seeds and grain used as cereal, add any milk you are not allergic to (cow, soy, almond, rice, banana, coconut, cashew), dried or fresh fruits or soaked nuts, and sweetener if needed like honey, maple syrup, or rice syrup. You can also stock up on this homemade cereal by purchasing the sunflower seeds or buckwheat groats in bulk. Several pound bags will last weeks and months. You can also overroast it.

Food Allergies Cause Gut Reactions

Hidden food allergies are a major cause of gut symptoms. Because every food has over a dozen mechanisms by which it can cause symptoms, I will teach you how to diagnose the most common ones.

For example, in reviewing the food allergies of the last one hundred people who initially came to me with gastrointestinal symptoms, I found the majority of them were triggered by foods such as milk, wheat, ferments and sugar—not brown rice, carrots, or peas. Thus it makes perfect sense to start our discussion wiht the most commonly implicated food allergy culprits.

Milk allergy is definitely one of the top unsuspected causes of gastrointestinal symptoms. In allergic individuals, it is a chief cause of constant nasal congestion and recurrent ear and sinus infections. For the person with irritable bowel syndrome (IBS), another mechanism of milk intolerance predominates. Some folks are born with a deficiency of lactase, the disaccharide enzyme that breaks down milk sugar, or lactose, into two simple sugars, glucose and galactose. Other folks can slowly develop a deficiency of the enzyme over many years, which I will discuss further in Chapter 5.

Those with lactase deficiency cannot properly digest lactose, so every time any dairy product is ingested, gas, bloating, pain, mucus, and diarrhea can occur—either right away or hours later. To confuse the diagnosis, some folks have only a partial deficiency of the enzyme, allowing them to digest some dairy foods where bacterial fermentation has partially digested the lactose. Hence, they tolerate some yogurts and cheeses or special milks with enzymes in them to digest lactose.

The simple solution is to have no dairy for one week, then spend a day consuming milk, ice cream, cream sauces, sour cream, cheeses, and other dairy foods that you love. Within less than forty-eight hours your gut will tell you whether you have a lactase deficiency. Meanwhile, avoid artificial creamers, since they all seem to have hydrogenated oils in them, which translates into trans fatty acids that promote premature aging of all body cells, including gut cells.

Milk and wheat vie for the top position among foods that cause gut symptoms. Like milk, wheat has many mechanisms to damage the gut with. The resulting most serious condition is called celiac disease, coeliac disease, celiac sprue, or gluten enteropathy.

Celiac victims exhibit a spectrum of symptoms from gas, bloating, indigestion, mucus, depression, or pain, to serious destruction of the gut lining. Here with the wall of the small intestine severely stripped bare of its microscopic absorptive fingerlike projections called villi, serious life-threatening malabsorption and weight loss can occur. Folks with destroyed gut linings can die if diagnosis and treatment are not instituted in time. And because this type of allergy can occur at any time, it is often unrecognized.

Unfortunately, once folks develop a sensitivity to gluten, one of the proteins in wheat, they also must avoid other grains that contain gluten, including rye, oats, and barley. Some folks are so seriously ill that they must avoid all grains. If even a trace of wheat contaminates the air of the grain mill where their other "safe" grains come from, for example, their corn or rice, that can also trigger a gluten reaction.

For such folks with severe gluten sensitivity, the mere stirring of one of their safe foods with a spoon that has been in a wheat dish can start the reaction of denuding the gut wall of its absorptive surfaces, or villi, as well. Once a person has suspected gluten enteropathy, he or she must religiously avoid all gluten for six months in order to heal the gut. One tiny indiscretion, such as a taste of something containing wheat, can start the whole vicious process over again, requiring six more months to heal the gut.

There is a blood test for the two common antibodies that cause celiac disease—the antigluten and antigliadin antibodies—but they are not foolproof. The only foolproof test is avoidance. If you start to feel better when avoiding grains, then keep at it. For a more detailed discussion, I refer you to my book *Wellness Against All Odds*. Anything that serious requires that you become an expert in it yourself.

Avoiding grains is not as easy as giving up just all breads, cookies, pasta, pretzels, biscuits, cakes, crackers, and other obvious sources of grains. You must be aware of hidden sources like meatloafs, gravies, breaded fish, and the grains used in whiskey.

Some folks actually have hidden food addictions to foods like milk, wheat, sugar, alcohol, or coffee that drive them to stay constantly fueled with that food. Because there are actual opioid receptors in the brain and in the gut that make folks crave a food, they will go out of their way to make sure they have a constant infusion of it. Likewise, withdrawal symptoms, like headache, agitation, or nausea, make avoidance difficult for the few days that they last.

Figuring Out Your Food Allergies

The rare food diagnostic diet shows you how to identify allergenic foods that trigger your symptoms and what foods you can eat. While on the diet, you just don't eat foods that you normally eat at least once every four days. So out goes milk, wheat, citrus, corn, chocolate, coffee, potato, soy, and more, depending upon your normal fare.

There is no perfect diet for everyone, for no two people have the same food allergies. You may be lucky in deciding that you do indeed eat a lot of dairy or processed foods and by avoiding them, your symptoms will disappear. On the other hand, where there is one food allergy, there are usually many, so it can become much more difficult to ferret out all the culprits—in which case the diet is the easiest means of doing so.

For example, a surgeon friend of mine had gas, bloating, and pain under his right ribs every time he ate. He and his colleagues were convinced that his symptoms were due to gallbladder disease. Thus, he did what surgeons do best, resorted to surgery. Imagine his frustration when he found he had just as much pain after the surgery as he had before the removal of his gall-bladder. He was more frustrated to find that when he followed the rare food diagnostic diet, all his symptoms disappeared. What looked like gallblad-der disease, even to a surgeon, was food allergy in disguise.

So, depending upon your symptoms, there are many options in terms of finding which food sensitivities you may have. If you have gastritis with ir-ritation and burning of the stomach, esophagitis, or suspect you have ul-cers, obviously you want to eliminate the c-r-a-p (coffee, cigarettes, alcohol, aspirin, processed foods—the junk). If you have gas, bloating, and diarrhea, why not start simply by avoiding milk, wheat, and sugar? If, as my surgeon friend, you have symptoms of gallbladder disease, then cut out the fats you normally eat for two weeks as well.

On the other hand if you have lost weight or have colitis with blood in the stool or abominal pain, you may need to follow a rigid gluten-free diet (special biopsies can be used to diagnose colitis if you want proof before a trial). Or your answer may lie in the next few chapters.

WHAT ABOUT BLOOD TESTS TO DIAGNOSE FOOD ALLERGIES?

There are many antibody tests that can show whether you make specific antibodies to foods. They are expensive and only test one or two of the mechanisms (types of an-tibodies) at a time. They are not fully accurate, because there are false negatives (you can be allergic to the food by another mechanism, such as enzyme deficiency, while the test looks for immunoglobulin G [IgG] antibody to the food) and false positives (you can make antibodies to the food but eating it does not produce symptoms). Therefore, the diagnostic diet is cheaper and more reliable. And it can be done in sim-ple stages, as eliminating then reintroducing one food at a time, or several at once.

The Diagnostic Diet

The diagnostic diet is one of the least expensive and most accurate ways to diagnose your hidden food allergies. The principle is to eat no foods for two weeks that you normally eat once a week or more frequently. So every-thing that you eat at least every week is out, including all dairy, wheat, eggs, corn, citrus, coffee, chocolate, and so on.

What is left? Brown rice, poached non–farm-raised fish, and steamed vegetables, or more unusual grains like millet, quinoa, amaranth, or teff. (For directions on how to prepare whole grains, greens, and beans, I refer you to *Macro Mellow,* a book by my allergy assistant and friend of over twenty years, Shirley Gallinger.) Think also of less frequently eaten veggies like squash, collards, kale, rutabaga, turnips, kohlrabi, or cassava. On the diet, breakfast could consist of soaked buckwheat groats and sunflower seeds with dried figs; snacks could consist of cashews or almond butter on rice cakes. For lunch, why not try homemade squash soup, nut flour muffins, or canned ocean salmon with homemade mayonnaise in an avocado.

Eat nothing that comes prepackaged with a list of ingredients, but only pure unadulterated foods of whole grains, greens and beans, seeds, and weeds. All multi-ingredient items should be homemade. Many types of meats, particularly wild game, would be fine. Free-range buffalo meat is now commonly available, as are some lamb and beef, all raised without antibiotics or pesticides. The animals are allowed to graze and choose their foods instinctively; they are not forced to eat commercial feed.

Animals have wonderful instincts about what to eat. They don't hobble around the pasture sucking down pain pills or sporting Ace bandages. If they don't feel well, they fast or forage for vegetation that heals them. And they certainly do not break the rules of nature (unless forced to for self-preservation), like having cows eat the ground-up carcasses of dogs or sheep, the cause of mad cow disease. In addition, the value of exercise and live food straight from the pasture cannot be duplicated by dead, ground-up, moldy, pesticided grains laced with additives to promote growth in animals that spend their days standing in a cramped stall or dung-filled feed lot. You may not always be able to find organic meat, fish, and fowl, but naturally raised, pastured, or free-range are the next best choice.

Monitor whether you suffer from withdrawal in the first few days, then see if you start feeling better by the end of the first week. At the end of two weeks, add back the foods you miss the most one day at a time and see what happens. Many people are surprised by the symptoms they get from their favorite and commonly eaten foods.

Bear in mind that there is a whole spectrum of gut diseases. For some people on the diet, getting off the junk and eating real foods will be curative in and of itself. Others will have food allergies or intolerances. Others still will discover where their symptoms come from with the information contained in the next chapters. For many people, too, the gut is so damaged that they will need to use some of the nontoxic, nonprescription remedies discussed in Chapter 6 to heal it before they can even tell what foods bother them. For other people, whose guts are already too torn up and irritated, only blended or juiced meals will be tolerated.

Should you have IBS, conquering it can be as simple as eliminating dairy. And even that may not be a life sentence. As you will learn, many gut enzymes, even lactase, can be produced again, once the gut wall is healed and lactase-splitting probiotics (as discussed in Chapter 4) are introduced. It is only medical professionals who, because they rarely seek the cause, usually think these conditions are incurable. Likewise, food allergies are not necessarily forever. Once you learn how to heal the gut and use enzymes (as discussed in Chapter 5), many food allergies disappear, including coeliac disease.

Simply by avoiding milk, wheat, sugars, and other processed foods for one to two weeks and identifying food allergies, may be all it takes to heal the gut. For other people, the easy-to-follow diet spelled out in the next chapter will suffice. This diet is designed to accomplish two goals: avoiding common antigens, or foods that cause gut symptoms, and avoiding foods that feed invading yeast organisms in the gut.

Other people, as those with severe spastic colitis, Crohn's disease (regional enteritis), or ulcerative colitis, may need to rotate foods religiously and strictly avoid commonly eaten foods at the same time. For half a century now, studies have shown what medicine still continues to ignore; that a hidden food allergy is both curative and causitive in a majority of folks with the most severe form of intestinal disease (Jones, Riordan, Rowe, Brostoff, Bently, Hyzms).

There are many things that you will learn as you proceed through this book that you may not think (or at least you hope) will not pertain to you. You may even try out some of the dietary suggestions and feel no difference in your overall health. But don't lose sight of the fact that as long as you have yet to diagnose what causes your symptoms, you may very well continue to suffer them. More about this later, but don't give up on yourself in the meantime as you enjoy your journey through the curable causes of most gut symptoms.

Last, but not least, when trying to figure out hidden food allergies, remember you must be aware of your diet type. Just as you cannot put diesel fuel in a gasoline engine and expect it to run well, we humans have different types of engines. Some folks have vegan-type engines. They thrive on grains, greens, and beans. To complicate matters more, some people tend more toward live or raw foods, while others need everything cooked.

Other folks are carnivores. They need high-quality protein at every meal. They must have eggs, salmon, or leftover meat for breakfast. Lunch and dinner must contain meat in some form as well. There are different subdivisions of this type of person as well: the slow and fast metabolizers. The slow metabolizers need fewer meats and leaner cuts, while the fast metabolizers include folks who thrive on more fat than usual and who don't gain weight or have high cholesterol. They have the metabolism to handle it and, if given free choice, go for the fat.

The point is that in designing your personal diet, you must be aware of whether you are a carnivore or vegan. For if you are doing a trial of singular foods, you will get very unhappy, weak, and dissatisfied if you do not have enough protein for too long. Make sure you incorporate sufficient protein into your diet plan; in effect, from 10 to 40 percent of your total diet, depending on your body type.

The Three Musketeers: Macronutrients

Let's look at the three types of macronutrients. First there are carbohydrates that come from fruits and vegetables, grains, and beans, with the proviso that you avoid white sugar and white bleached flour. Next, we have the proteins, supplying the amino acid building blocks of muscle and hormones. When avoiding red meat grown on feed lots with hormones, pesticides, and processed animal feed, we can turn to grains, beans, nuts and seeds to get our protein. Last are the fats, which we all try to avoid but frankly can't live without. The truth is we need all three of the components just mentioned—carbohydrates, proteins, and fats—but it is the balance and quality that counts.

Should you find out that you are more suited to be a vegan versus a carnivore or an omnivore (one who eats a little of both meat and vegetables), you can determine the balance that is best for your body. Remember, if you try to give your diesel engine gasoline, your engine will come to a grinding halt. In Table 6 I've listed the best and worst sources for macronutrients to help you begin to phase out from your diet the disease-producing processed foods you now may consume.

Obviously, since opposites attract and carnivores are usually married to vegans, it can be lethal to cram a vegan meal down a carnivore's throat and vice versa. When I was rapidly healing over twenty ailments with the macrobiotic diet, my carnivore husband lost thirty pounds in one month on it. Much marital discord and many divorces have resulted from failure to realize that just because one person feels fantastic on a diet does not mean that everyone should. Instead, learn to switch the proportions. You can cook what the carnivore needs for a meal, but give him or her just tiny amounts of grains, greens, and beans. Whereas the vegan may not chose to indulge in some of the meat that the carnivore is served but has huge portions of the grains, greens, and beans. This is an absolute must in keeping marital harmony and health. So, if you are a vegan, don't get on your high horse and turn up your nose at the carnivores. Your emotional health will benefit even as your physical health flowers.

Table 6. Sources of Macronutrients

Best source	*Worse source* (once a week, or never have unless homemade)
Carbohydrates Fresh, raw, or steamed vegetables; local fresh fruit; whole grains, or whole-grain breads and whole-grain pastas; beans	**Carbohydrates** Foods with long cooking times; canned reheated, or frozen vegetables; commercially prepared cookies, white breads, pasta, cake, candy, pop tarts, pretzels, jam, pie, bagels, chips, sugar
Proteins Organic and naturally raised meat and fowl; jellied tongue; heart; sardines; cod liver, Alaskan salmon; unfarmed (if available) fresh fish; tuna; beans; free-range chicken; raw milk or organic cheeses; organic yogurt; processed cheese;	**Proteins** Cold cuts; fast food; burgers; ravioli; sausages; fried fish sticks; artificial dairy products like cottage cheese and poor-quality grocery-store yogurt with sugar; milk
Fats Cold-pressed organic oils; seeds; nuts; organic fermented dairy, as in cottage cheese or yogurt; butter (if you are not lactase deficient or have corrected lactase deficiency)	**Fats** Mayonnaise; margarine; grocery-store hydrogenated oils, especially soybean; salted, roasted nuts; processed cheeses

Are You Eating a Rainbow Each Day?

The call to action? Eat a rainbow diet each day. The more whole, raw, or slightly steamed vegetables you have, the more your meals will be power-packed with healing nutrients. Organic is best. Next is fresh, local produce from the farmers' market. The further away produce comes from, the greater the chance that pesticides were used to prevent bugs from devouring the vegetables on their journey. In general, the least healthy produce comes from outside the country—for many countries do not have restrictive rules regarding the use of pesticides outlawed in the United States years ago. At the same time, it's wishful thinking to believe that workers applying the pesticides can always, and always do, read the English warnings on the pesticide packages.

Color is where the healing parts of foods are hidden, so make sure your plate is colorful: red, yellow, blue, purple, orange, and green. (See Table 8.) In fact, play a game and see how many ways you can think of for getting foods that contain these natural colors, nature's richest source of carotenoids and other disease-fighting phytochemicals. The more rainbow foods

Table 7. Macronutrient Proportions for Diet Types

Diet Type	Carbohydrate	Protein	Fat
Carnivore	30%	40%	30%
Omnivore	50%	30%	20%
Vegan	75%	15%	15%
Raw vegan	80%	10%	10%

you eat, the less room there will be on your plate for dead, colorless foods that are stripped of their nautral healing nutrients.

In case you are confused about how much to eat, follow the two to four colors per meal rule. Since colored veggies and fruits contain the majority of healing phytonutrients (plant-based nutrients), you'll want to build your meals around these colors, factoring in other foods that enable you to complement your diet type.

For example, the carnivore can now add his or her meat and fat (butter for veggies), and the vegan can add his or her whole grains and beans. However, in the early stages of identifying your food allergies, start with mono meals (one food at a meal) as discussed. Once you determine a particular food does not provoke symptoms, you can add another food. With time, you should have a balanced meal of whole foods, not one bogged down with processed foods that are nutrient-depleted and loaded with chemicals that are difficult to digest.

It May Not Be What You Are Eating, But What's Eating You

We joke about how a certain person or situation gives us ulcers, and even hospitalized patients under severe stress have proven the role of stress in causing ulcers. Here is where your spirituality can rescue you as you incorporate forgiveness and intentional acts of kindness into your total plan for self-healing. Learn to replace worry with constructive planning and a brighter view of the world.

The body's nervous system has two phases: the sympathetic and the parasympathetic. The sympathetic nervous system is referred to as the fight-or-flight-system. It readies us for survival via active defense or sudden flight. So most of the blood flow is directed toward muscles. But you don't need to be threatened by a tiger to throw your nervous system into the sympathetic phase. A hectic day at the office can leave you in the same mode. Anger, anxiety, and tension can leave the neck, cranial, and back muscles knotted up and aching. And so can the stomach be left in knots.

Table 8. Ideas for the Rainbow Diet

Red: peppers, tomatoes, watermelon, raspberries, strawberries, beets, red raspberries

Yellow: squash, peppers, sweet potatoes

Orange: carrots, squash, peppers, sweet potatoes

Green: greens (lettuces, collards, kale, watercress), melons, scallions, parsley, brussel sprouts, broccoli, squash

White: onions, potatoes, cauliflower, squash, mushrooms

Purple/Blue: red cabbage, turnips, kohlrabi, radishes, beets, plums, grapes, blueberries

Solutions:
- rainbow diet (see how many colors you can get of living or lightly steamed foods)
- carrot juice 1–3 times a day
- crudités (artfully cut carrots, celery, scallions, radishes, cauliflower, broccoli, and other vegetables) before every dinner to replace snacks of chips, pretzels, and other dead and processed foods. Make healthful sauerkraut blended with homemade mayonnaise with herbs or humus dips
- cut dead food (breads, meats, pastas, sodas, processed foods) to less than 20%

The parasympathetic nervous system allows for body maintenance replacements and repair functions, like digestion, hormone secretions, daily repair, and special healing. If we mentally keep ourselves in sympathetic overdrive, we cheat ourselves out of proper digestion and healing.

In a Nutshell

With a monotonous diet, such as one that includes wheat at every meal (in breads, cereals, or pasta), we can overwhelm our capacities to recognize specific antibodies, prompting the body to produce antibodies—yes, even to wheat—that then turn on the body itself, denuding the absorptive surface of the small intestine. What to do? Eat a varied diet to provide a wider base of nutrients.

Still, there are more ways in which our food choices cause any number of symptoms. Food allergy or intolerance can also trigger the production of antibodies to the food of concern, which causes immediate rejection, such as vomiting after eating peanuts and nausea from the outpouring of excess acid needed to digest the huge amounts and multiple food combinations we sometimes eat. Or the body can stop making enough digestive enzymes for a number of reasons, including mineral and other nutrient deficiencies.

Food itself may not be as problematic as the chemicals added to food and the natural nutrients taken out of food during processing. As I have discussed, food additives can also trigger gut symptoms as potential side effects. At the same time, nearly every drug you take causes digestive symptoms, with aspirin and nonsterodial anti-inflammatory medications like Motrin, Aleve, Advil, and Voltaren having the potential of causing severe gastric pain and even hemorrhaging.

Finally, the atmosphere in which we eat can induce us to secrete digestive enzymes peacefully or to shut the entire process down, setting the stage for massive indigestion minutes or hours later. *Bottom line:* The foods and drugs we consume on a daily basis have a profound impact on the health of the gut.

The simplest solution is to limit each meal to one or two food types and observe how you feel. Your diet is dependent upon specific foods. Whether dairy, wheat, sugar, processed foods, alcohol, or coffee, eliminate that particular food for a week and then consume a large amount. You'll know quickly enough if any of the foods you've just eaten are culprits.

And if you have a more serious condition involving severe pain, bleeding, or weight loss, I assume you have had a workup to rule out cancer and have a label like Crohn's disease or ulcerative colitis. But be sure you have done a trial gluten-free diet even if you have negative antigluten antibodies and antigliadin antibodies. In fact, for conditions that serious, dairy, sugar, and grain-free diets may be the only way to heal. Regardless of what you may need to avoid, most intolerances and allergies don't last forever. They can disappear once you have healed.

Since dairy, grains, sugars, and processed foods are the most common causes of indigestion, the simplest approach would be the diet as given in the next chapter.

CHAPTER 3

Curing the Most Commonly Missed Cause of Gut Disease

Candida: The Great Masquerader

Do you stash Gummi Bears or candy bars in your desk? Are you a closet cookie monster? Are you obsessed with sweets? If so, you may unknowingly harbor yeasts that are gobbling up your sugars before you can use them. These hidden gremlins in the gut give the telltale sign of bloating and indigestion after meals, especially when you must let out your belt or plan on wearing looser clothes than you used to for any particular meal.

Of all the viruses, bacteria, and parasites I've treated in over a quarter of a century, none holds a candle to *Candida albicans* and the secret damage this supposedly harmless yeast can do. Even though Candida can cause symptoms that mimic more diseases than all the rest of the uninvited guests to the body, it is still presumed by the medical majority to be a normal part of our intestinal flora. Doctors may even argue that it is harmless unless you are in an extremely compromised state, such as end-stage cancer. But unsuspected *Candida albicans* is one of the biggest reasons why some people just never get better.

Although *Candida albicans* is one of the more common types of yeast and we normally house small amounts of it in our intestines, if the delicate balance between Candida and the other bugs in the gut is tipped, Candida grows rampantly, which can produce over one hundred different symptoms, beginning with the gut.

The Many Causes of Candida Outbreak

Taking antibiotics that kill off hundreds of types of bacteria but not yeasts, is the most common way to cause a Candida outbreak. With no competition and with Candida leading the way, the yeasts grow wildly, taking control of the gut. Diets high in sugar will also enhance the yeast outbreak as can medications like prednisone, birth control pills, and other synthetic estrogens.

Unfortunately, synthetic estrogens are not limited to medication, but can silently sneak into our bodies from toxic chemicals called estrogen mimics used in plastic bottles holding soda, baby formula, and bottled water, as well as from plastic wraps for candy bars and supermarket meats and vegetables. In addition, estrogen mimics can enter our bodies from the pesticides that continue to contaminate our food, air, and water (Jobling).

Undiagnosed, It Mimics Any Symptom

Once Candida takes over the gut, it inflames the gut wall provoking much of the gas, bloating, indigestion, alternating diarrhea and constipation, or pain that you may suffer. If the yeast inflames the lower esophagus or stomach, you have burning and heartburn. If the lining of the small intestine is inflamed, carrier, or transport, proteins are damaged, making it more difficult for the gut to absorb vitamins and minerals—with mysterious fatigue and new infections the possible result. Now, with the gut inflamed, putrifactive toxins from the contents of the bowel leak into the bloodstream, prompting aches and pains all over (mysterious fibromyalgia), as well as damaging local nerves in the gut, which leads to constipation.

Because the inflamed gut can leak large food particles that the immune system has never encountered before, an antibody attack is mounted against them. Suddenly the innocent host of Candida (you!) has food allergies to all sorts of foods that never bothered you before.

But food allergies are only the beginning. As Candida inflames the gut wall, where half the body's detoxification system lies, you may find yourself reacting to perfumes, smoke, cleansers, shopping malls, offices, and chemicals in the environment with runny nose, headache, brain fog, depression, fatigue, dizziness, or aching all over, with pains mysteriously migrating from one spot to another.

These are but a sampling of the symptoms that can occur seemingly overnight or that can build slowly over months. As time passes, more symptoms may develop with each week. Despite volumes of scientific studies, for some inexplicable reason, most of the medical community still refuses to acknowledge that Candida can do all the damage it does. (For a more in-depth explanation of this phenomenon, see my book *Depression Cured At Last!)*

Begin with a Suspicion or Diagnosis

For those who are sick of being sick and who wish to determine if they suffer from an outbreak of Candida, forge ahead. Within one month of following the strict program below, you should sense a convincing difference in the way you feel and act. For those who want to play it safe and start with a medical diagnosis, have your doctor order a special stool test to determine if Candida is growing in your gut. (See Chapter 7.) Merely get a prescription for the test, call the 800 number of the lab, have the kit sent to you, put your stool in it according to directions, mail it back, and wait for the results.

If you do want a medical diagnosis, be sure not to treat the yeast for at least one week prior to giving the stool sample, or you may lessen the amount of Candida found, or the lab may not find any at all—the test itself is not precisely definitive. In my experience, only 5 to 10 percent of patients tested received negative results. The only way we surmised these folks had Candida was when they felt 100 percent better while on the yeast program.

Of course, there is absolutely no harm in doing the yeast program, so you might decide to go for the program without the test. Nonetheless, many of us prefer to know what is being treated, especially if you happen to have a huge amount of Candida or it is a particularly resistant form that requires special treatment beyond what you can do on your own.

Caveats

A few items you should be aware of that could sabotage your good intentions.

1. As most people start to learn how to rid themselves of yeasts, they get overwhelmed with self-pity and worry about having to deny themselves a few foods for a short while. Remember, this is not a life sentence. It is a diagnostic and therapeutic trial of one to six months. Once you are well, you can eat anything.
2. As yeasts are killed off, they let loose with their toxins and wastes. This can make you, the host, feel worse than you ever have. It's called

a die-off reaction and rarely lasts more than a day or two. The good part, of course, is that it reaffirms just how much you needed the program. If symptoms last more than a week, something else is wrong. Stop the program and see your doctor. To minimize and possibly avoid die-off, simply take a laxative before you start the program. By hoeing out the gut, you will reduce the number of organisms present and there will be fewer symptom-producing toxins released.

To hoe out the gut, take one to two tablespoons of milk of magnesia (available in any grocery or pharmacy) or an herbal gut-purifiying laxative like the two-stage Nature's Pure Body Program (Pure Body Institute). Take two to four tablets of the colon-cleansing bottle portion and four to eight tablets of the herbal body purification portion one to three times a day for two to fifteen days.

CANDIDA TIPS

• Do you feel better after taking a large dose of vitamin B_1 or thiamine? Some species of Candida make thiaminase, an enzyme to break down this energy vitamin before it gets absorbed. So be sure to take Alli-thiamine (Ecologic Formulas), a better-absorbed fat-soluble form (50 milligrams thiamine tetrahydrofurfuryl disulfide), one or two times a day.

• After years of fighting Candida, some people have grown resistant forms of it. *Candida tropicalis,* for example, resists Nystatin, a powder prescribed to kill yeast. To avoid undue difficulties here, diagnose the problem before tackling it with the nonprescription yeast fighters detailed later on in combination with a sytemic antifungal like ketoconazole (Nizoral) or fluconazole (Diflucan).

• When were you last really well? Have you taken a full course of antibiotics in the five years before that, say for acne, cystitis, prostatitis, root canal, or repeated bouts of sinusitis? If so, you may never get well until you reduce the Candida to normal levels.

Your Anti-Candida Program to Beat the Yeast

Conquering yeasts and all the symptoms they cause is a multistage pyramid. You can take all the time you feel you need between stages, from one day to several weeks. The steps are quite simple:

1. Empty the gut
2. Start the yeast-free, mold-free, sugar-free diet
3. Start the probiotics (the good bugs like acidophilus, etc.)
4. Start other nonprescription yeast fighters (like garlic, etc.)

If this is not sufficient, you will need to enlist the help of your physician:

5. Start prescription Nystatin
6. Start prescription Nizoral, Diflucan, or others (as indicated by culture)
7. Do repeat culture to determine if yeast has been eradicated
8. See your doctor to determine causes and course for getting rid of any remaining symptoms

Yeasts Can Make You Drunk Without Drinking

There is one other aspect to Candida that most are unfamiliar with. As a living organism, Candida must rid itself of toxins. I refer more specifically to acetaldehyde, a Candida toxin that some folks may have problems with. In those who do not metabolize and excrete toxins as quickly and efficiently as they should, acetaldehyde can back up, causing a host of confusing symptoms. In fact, acetaldehyde is the same chemical that backs up in us if we have too much alcohol to drink. In this regard, one doesn't have to drink any alcohol at all to get the auto-brewery syndrome. With acetaldehyde, the gut bugs will make their own alcohol-like compounds.

In addition to having gas, bloating, indigestion, such folks can appear drunk and disoriented. Or they can have severe mood swings, depression, or even mania. In addition to gut and brain symptoms, acetaldehyde stimulates the chemistry behind cravings, making the very folks who need them the least crave sugars, alcohol, and ferments.

You should also know that, along with Candida, other fungi and organisms, or an inability to properly digest sugars that then contribute to a general imbalance of organisms, encouraging some to ferment, can all trigger auto-brewery syndrome. To quell auto-brewery syndrome, simply fulfill the regimen to eradicate Candida. Thanks to the work of England's Dr. Keith Eaton, studies show that for the majority of folks with unwanted yeasts in the gut, the following diet will clear their symptoms. So let's see what that diet entails.

Candida-Killing Diet

Are you ready to do the Candida yeast-free diet to see just how good you can feel? Then let's start by learning the foods you must avoid and the foods you can eat freely.

This diet does not count calories or limit portions, so please feel free to eat all the safe foods that you need to satisfy your appetite. There are certain foods you must strictly avoid, but there are many wonderful foods that you can enjoy. After you learn the no-no's, you can dive right into some unusual but great-tasting meals.

Foods You Must Strictly Avoid

Yeast Foods

Yeast (leavening) in all forms, yeast-raised breads, rolls, and pastries. This includes all fresh and frozen bagels, breads, biscuits, buns, and rolls. Also avoid all edible fungi (mushrooms). *Mold, yeast, mushroom,* and *fungus* are all terms relating to the yeast problem. Things that have been fermented, aged, pickled, yeasted, malted, risen, and even leftovers can harbor mold antigens that the body recognizes as belonging to or looking similar to Candida. When it attacks, you have symptoms.

Alcohol

You must strictly avoid all fermented beverages such as wine, beer, whiskey, brandy, gin, rum, vodka, and other fermented liquors and liqueurs.

Prepared Drinks

Also avoid fermented beverages such as apple cider, root beer, and all soft drinks. Coffees and teas of all types, including herb teas, must also be avoided, except organic Chinese or Japanese green tea.

Condiments and Commercial Salad Dressings

Other ferments include mustard, ketchup, Worcestershire sauce, soy sauce, pickles, pickled relishes, green and black olives, sauerkraut, horseradish, all types of vinegar, and all vinegar-containing foods such as commercially prepared mayonnaise and salad dressings.

Sugar

Sugar and sugar-containing foods (sucrose, fructose, maltose, lactose, glycogen, glucose, mannitol, sorbitol, galactose, monosaccharides, and polysaccharides) should be avoided. Other forms of sugar are honey, molasses, maple syrup, maple sugar, date sugar, turbinado sugar, rice syrup, and barley malt syrup. You must learn to read all package labels to see what is really hidden in there. Do not use aspartame (trade names Equal or Nutrasweet) or saccharin. (The warning on saccharin products reads "Use of this product may be hazardous to your health. This product contains saccharin, which has been determined to cause cancer in laboratory animals."

This warning oddly enough does not appear on over-the-counter nonprescription medications that also contain saccharin. Are they exempt?)

Safe Sugar Substitute

There is only one sweetener that is safe for a person fighting Candida: stevia. The leaf of a small shrub that has been used for over one hundred years by native populations, the herb stevia is ten to fifteen times sweeter than common sugar from sugar cane. Stevia is used in many countries and appears to be extremely safe for regular use as a sweetener in drinks, dips, dressings, and in baked goods—although it does not brown baked goods as regular sugar will. Stevia is available in many health food stores in either liquid or powdered form. If you are unable to find it locally, you can call Environmental Health Link at (419) 659-5541 for a source nearest to you.

Cheese

All cheeses contain molds. This includes prepared foods with cheese added, such as Velveeta Macaroni and Cheese, cheese snacks and crackers, plus buttermilk, sour cream, and yogurt products. Almost all dairy products, except for pure unsalted butter and ghee, contain high levels of yeast. Be sure to read all labels, as dairy products are often hidden in prepared foods. If you find yourself wondering, "On this diet can I eat . . . such and such?" remind yourself of one motto: When in doubt, leave it out.

Processed Foods

It is also very important to avoid all processed and packaged foods. They usually contain refined sugar products and many other hidden ingredients derived from yeasts, such as B vitamin fortification. As well, most prepared or processed foods are so old they are bound to have mold antigens.

Malt products must also be avoided, including malted-milk drinks, cereals, and candy, and as also found in the ingredients of many processed foods. You really do have to read all labels carefully. In fact, if something has a list of ingredients you probably don't want it anyway. You want pure, unadulterated, natural, whole foods with live enzymes that can kill Candida and fortify the intestines. Other items to avoid are all processed and/or smoked meats, such as sausages, hot dogs, corned beef, and pastrami.

Fruits

Because fruits are high in the sugar that yeasts thrive on, you will need to avoid all fruits until you kill sufficient yeast. Many folks have been amazed at how one piece of fruit eaten before the right time in the program caused a reduplication of symptoms—after they had been so free of them. Raw vegetables are just as healthful, but won't trigger yeasts to flourish.

Avoid dried and candied fruits, such as raisins, apricots, dates, prunes, and figs.

Likewise, avoid all fruit juices that are canned, bottled, or frozen. Freshly prepared juices and whole fresh fruits sometimes may be used after the first three weeks on the strict diet, but only after you are totally free of symptoms.

Since many miss breads and fruits the most, you can choose whichever you please when it comes time to do a trial of adding foods back into your diet.

Medications

Avoid the many drugs that encourage yeast. If your doctor wishes to treat you with antibiotics, be sure there is very good evidence for him or her to do so. If the problem is really allergic or viral, antibiotics do not help. If you must take an antibotic, stay on the diet and keep taking probiotics like *Lactobacillus acidophilus,* but stop taking Nystatin and Nizoral to avoid fostering the growth of fungi that could become resistant to them. If possible, try to avoid all cortisone-type drugs as well as oral contraceptives and synthetic estrogens.

Foods You May Eat Freely

Try to find organic produce when possible, otherwise choose local or naturally grown produce, without added pesticides or chemicals. Wash all produce thoroughly before using. In terms of meat and fowl, after organic, free-range, naturally raised, or pastured is next best. It is tough to find non-farm-raised fish these days, and the contamination in some popular fishing waters rules them out. The more you know about the source of your food, the better. An asterisk (*) denotes that the recipe follows.

Group I Animal

Meat: beef, veal, lamb, pork, rabbit, venison, buffalo, and any game animals.

Poultry: chicken, Cornish hen, duck, goose, turkey, and eggs (preferably free-range, preferably organic).

Fish and Seafood: all foods from the water are fine if not breaded. Try to avoid farmed.

Group II Vegetables, Unlimited

BE SURE ALL VEGETABLES ARE WASHED WELL BEFORE EATING TO GET RID OF SURFACE YEASTS OR MOLDS. Because vegetables have an abundance of healing factors in them you can use the space after each one to note some of the more enticing ways to prepare them or where your favorite recipes are found to help you use more of each item.

Artichoke, globe
Artichoke, Jerusalem
Asparagus
Beets
Broccoli
Brussels sprouts
Cabbage (green, red, Chinese, savoy)
Carrots
Cauliflower
Celery
Celery root
Cucumber
Eggplant
Garlic (excellent for fighting Candida)
Greens: All lettuces, beet greens, bok choy, chives, collards, dandelion, kale, mustard, parsley, spinach, turnip, and watercress
Jicama
Kohlrabi
Okra
Onion (in all forms): Bermuda, pearl, Spanish, sweet, red, leeks, scallions, shallots, white, and yellow cooking
Parsley root
Parsnips
Pea pods
Peppers (sweet and hot)
Radishes (all types)
Rutabaga
String beans (green, yellow wax, Italian)
Summer squashes (all types)
Tomatoes (fresh only)
Turnips
Zucchini

Group III Vegetables, Limited

HIGHER IN CARBOHYDRATES, SO LIMIT TO ONE SMALL
SERVING PER MEAL FROM EACH OF THE THREE GROUPS (III a,
III b, III c)

III a: Starches

Sweet corn
Sweet potato/yam
Winter squash (acorn, butternut, etc.)
White potato

III b: Dried Beans and Peas (cooked)

Aduki
Black
Garbanzo (chickpea)
Lentil (green and red)
Kidney
Navy
Pinto
Soy (fresh green, dried beans, and tofu)
Green peas
Lima beans

III c: Whole Grains (The first six are grasses, the remaining ones are among the weed family)

Barley
Millet
Oats
Rice (brown and wild)
Rye
Wheat
Amaranth
Buckwheat
Quinoa
Teff

Broken Grains (Flours)

Your broken grains intake should be limited to one portion a day. Whole wheat or unbleached, organic unbromated white flour is best for quick breads, biscuits, or muffins made with aluminum-free Rumford baking powder or baking soda. Whole wheat pastas (bought in a health food store or through a health food catalog) are excellent choices. Commercial products which can safely be used are rice cakes, Ryvita Crispbread, and Kavali Crispbread (be sure to check ingredients as some do have yeast). Some German butcher shops in the United States have organic German flatbreads made with linseeds. Massa bread, made from sprouted grains, can often be found in health food stores and makes for a delicious treat. **REMEMBER: NO YEAST.** Bulgur, couscous, kamut, and spelt are wheat derivatives that have been processed and belong in this category. Wait a month after beginning the diet before using any of these foods.

Group IV: Seeds and Nuts

Choose smooth-skinned seeds and nuts only, like almonds and sunflower seeds. You want to avoid any ridges as in pecans and walnuts that hide mold.

Nuts

Almonds, homemade almond milk* or almond butter.* (They are more
   digestible if soaked overnight and peeled.)
Cashews, homemade cashew milk* or cashew butter*
Brazil nuts
Filberts

Seeds

Flax seed (linseed)
Pumpkin
Sesame, sesame tahini (butter), sesame milk
Sunflower
* See recipe section for nut, seed milk, and better butter recipes.

All seeds and nuts should be fresh, unroasted, unsalted, and preferably still in their shells. It is easy to roast seeds and nuts at home in either a skillet or the oven and doing so will kill any mold that might be present.

You can find these fresh nuts and seeds, as well as nut butters, at a good health food store or in mail-order catalogs. (See Resource Guide.)

Group V: Fats and Oils

Extra virgin olive oil is the best. An abundance of different flavors are available in ethnic, health food, and fine food stores.

Flax oil (organic, refrigerated, and dated) can also be found in health food stores. Do not heat flax oil: use in cold form only for salad dressing, in better butter*, or on cereals or vegetables. Because flax oil is over half omega-3 and less than one-fifth omega-6, long-term use can produce omega-6 deficiencies. That is why it is best to use flax on salads and to cook with olive oil (which contains omega-9 and a smidgen of omega-6). Although almond oil has a similar composition, the processing required to obtain it involves more stages. You can still get occasional omega-6 oils from organic cold-pressed corn, safflower, sesame, walnut, grape seed, or sunflower oils. Do not eat deep-fried foods, as the high temperature produces a change (trans fatty acids) in the oil that accumulates in and damages the body, promoting aging and disease. And don't be hoodwinked by words like polyunsaturated, for that is usually reserved for grocery-store oils that contain damaging trans fatty acids.

All oils should be cold pressed or expeller pressed, and are available at any health food store. Do not buy grocery-store oils, for nearly all are hydrogenated, having been exposed to very high temperatures to make them last. Hydrogenation not only destroys most of the nutritional content like vitamin E, but also creates harmful trans fatty acids. Avoid canola oil because it is genetically engineered seed, and avoid all soy oils, because over 80 percent are genetically engineered to be Round-up (an herbicide with carcinogenic potential) resistant. Therefore, they are usually heavily contaminated with this pesticide. Also avoid cottonseed oil, as cotton is not considered a food and can be laced with even more toxic pesticides.

Sesame oil
Safflower oil
Sunflower oil
Walnut oil

Other fats

Unsalted dairy butter
Better butter*
Homemade mayonnaise and salad dressings*

Group VI: Condiments

Sea salt
Black and white ground pepper

Fresh herbs (no dried herbs); even large supermarkets now often carry fresh herbs in their produce section. Basil, cilantro, and dill are favorites. Also experiment with replacing vinegars with lemon grass and lemon balm for tangy tastes in salad dressings.

Chopped parsley

Chopped scallions

Fresh lemon (OK in small amount needed for salad dressing)

Fresh lime (OK in small amount needed for salad dressing)

Preroasted sesame or sunflower seeds or nuts add zip to dishes, while grated and curled vegetables make great garnishes.

Save Cooking Liquor

Save the liquids left in the pan after you cook vegetables. This liquid is full of good nutrition and can be used as a hot or cold drink and can also become a soup or sauce base.

Snacks

Snacks need not be a problem. Crudités prepared from any of the unlimited vegetables, such as raw celery, carrot, sweet pepper, broccoli, cauliflower, cucumber, radishes, kohlrabi, fennel, and scallions and many more, make for tasty snacks. Homemade humus* and other bean, tofu, sauerkraut,* and seed dips and spreads can make your veggies a real treat. Prepared and kept in the refrigerator they are always ready when the yeast starts screaming "feed me."

Other safe snacks which are easy to carry while away from home are popcorn (freshly air-popped at home), hard-boiled eggs, cold chicken pieces, rice cakes with seed, bean, or nut spreads. Or create your own trail mix from various types of seeds and nuts; make them as organic as possible, and avoid the already-prepared ones roasted with sugar and salt. I'm sure you can come up with even more ideas to suit your tastes.

Seeds and nuts are a good way to satisfy real hunger. Please be sure to try the nut and seed milks as well. They taste sinfully good, and are the core of nutritious dessert toppings when you get well; for now they are another way to add more variety to your meals.

Sample Diet for One Week

These are only suggestions to get you started. I know there will be many who do not eat red meat and many who choose to eat no meat. Please feel free to substitute any fish or fowl for meat in any day's menu. If possible, try to find organic sources of animal food to avoid the antibiotics and hormones added by ranchers worldwide. We really don't need or want these items in our food, as they lower immune competence. When frying, use extra virgin olive oil and keep heat as low as you can. Never cook with flax, but use it raw.

Leftovers should be frozen if they will not be used the next day. Mold grows rapidly in food which is not frozen.

The more fresh vegetables you have at a meal the better; if they are raw, then all the better. If cooked, do them al dente, with a hollandaise or other sauce to improve family acceptance of two to four veggies per meal.

THE TIME TO GO SHOPPING IS NOW. BE PREPARED TO START YOUR YEAST-FREE, SUGAR-FREE, FERMENT-FREE ADVENTURE, AND HAVE "FUN FOODS" ON HAND LIKE NUTS, SO YOU ARE NOT TEMPTED TO CHEAT.

BON APPETIT!

SUNDAY

BREAKFAST   Eggs (any style)
Fried, sliced tomatoes with fresh herbs
Toasted rice cakes with homemade or organic nut butter
Hot water with lemon or flax seeds or sliced ginger root

LUNCH   Large chef salad with a variety of veggies with shrimp or tuna
Ferment-free flax oil and lemon dressing*
Rice cakes or yeast-free crackers or breads

DINNER   Baked chicken
Vegetables of choice from Group II (pick three or four)
One high carbohydrate vegetable from Group III such as Barley salad*
Water with lemon slice

SNACKS   Nuts or seeds
Crudités (carrot, celery, cucumber sticks, radishes)

MONDAY

BREAKFAST   Bowl of cooked brown rice with butter or flax oil
Sprinkle with nuts or seeds of choice
Hot water with lemon slice or fresh vegetable juice, like carrot
Sunday's leftover vegetables

LUNCH   Leftover cold chicken from Sunday dinner
Lightly steamed vegetables from Group II or raw vegetable salad
Nut butter on rice cakes
Bottled water
This lunch would be easy to carry to work, as would any raw salad that could also contain some cooked veggies marinated in herbs, oil and fresh lemon juice, topped with sardines or tuna. When selecting sardines, those packed in sild oil are best but hard to find. Next best is spring water. Do not get boneless or skinless sardines.

DINNER   Broiled beef steak or ground beef patty
Two vegetables from Group II
One vegetable or grain from Group III (a small baked potato would be fine)
Dinner salad with safe dressing if desired

SNACKS   Nut butter spread on celery stalks, scallions, cucumber, or carrot sticks

TUESDAY

BREAKFAST   Cooked hot oatmeal with almond milk* and sprinkles
Safe beverage of choice

LUNCH   Tuna salad with celery and onion, prepared with either oil and lemon or ferment-free mayonnaise*
Raw vegetables of choice from Group II, with or without humus or other bean dip
Rice cakes or crackers

Safe beverage of choice

Alaskan Salmon salad* is another lunch which is easy to carry to work.

DINNER   Broiled fish or pork chop
Vegetables of choice from Group II
One choice from Group III (bake extra potatoes)
Small dinner salad or vegetable slaw* with safe dressing

SNACKS   Seeds or nuts, raw vegetables with or without dip

WEDNESDAY

BREAKFAST   Eggs (any style)
Fried, sliced, leftover sweet potatoes
Cornmeal grits with butter
Hot water with lemon

LUNCH   Large chef salad with hard-boiled egg and shrimp or crab and safe dressing
Rice cakes or crackers or unyeasted bread, biscuit, or muffin*
Water with lemon

DINNER   Broiled lamb or veal chops
Two vegetables from Group II
One choice from Group II (bake extra squash)
Salad with safe dressing

SNACK   Sardines on rice cake or flatbread*
Seeds or nuts

THURSDAY

BREAKFAST   Hot whole buckwheat cereal or shredded wheat (no additives, no sugar)
Fried herbed squash patties
Nut milk and sprinkles*
Hot water with lemon

LUNCH   Homemade beef-barley-vegetable soup*
Raw veggies
Biscuits or flatbread*
Freeze leftover soup for Saturday lunch

DINNER   Turkey slices from small roast
Two vegetables from Group II
One choice from Group III
Dinner salad with safe dressing
Save slices of turkey for tomorrow's lunch

SNACKS   Raw vegetable sticks with avocado dip*
Seeds or nuts

FRIDAY

BREAKFAST   Hot oatmeal with butter and nuts or almond milk and sprinkles* or soup with extra diced carrots, celery, and chopped scallions
Hot water with lemon

LUNCH   Large chef salad with strips of turkey breast and safe dressing
Rice cakes or corn bread*
Pure water with lemon

DINNER   Broiled salmon with lemon and dill
Brown rice pilaf
Two vegetables from Group II
Cabbage and carrot slaw*

SNACKS   Crudités with safe dip

SATURDAY

BREAKFAST   Eggs (any style) or scrambled tofu with diced vegetables
Corn muffins*
Hot water with lemon

LUNCH   Rerun of beef-barley-vegetable soup
                 Plate of raw veggies (Group II) with humus*
                 Water with lemon juice

DINNER   Stir-fry with meat or fish of choice and
                 Choice of vegetables (Group II)
                 Over brown rice (Group III)
                 Dinner salad with safe dressing
                 Hot water with lemon

There you are—a whole week of nutritional, yeast-free, sugar-free, ferment-free menus. You can just keep repeating for another week or start planning your own. From this point on, you want a minimum of three large servings of raw veggies a day. Crudités, chef salad, multiveggie salad, cole slaw, and barley salad are great ways to accomplish this. Slaws can be made not only from thinly shredded cabbage, onion, and celery, but also carrots, broccoli (stems peeled and shredded), cauliflower, and other vegetables. Use your imagination.

When Can I Eat My Favorites Again?

After three to six weeks, if all is going well, you may want to do the yeast challenge and then the fruit challenge. But do not add foods until you are well. There is no point in going backward once you start healing.

The Fruit Challenge

After three weeks on your diet, if all is going well, you may try the fruit challenge. Initially, the safest fruits to try are bananas, apples, and strawberries; do not start with melons or watermelon as they are considered to be a moldy food.

Start with a banana, taking a small bite. If there is no reaction after ten minutes, take a second bite. If no reaction develops in the next hour, eat the rest of the banana. If you tolerate the banana without developing symptoms, you can test other fruits, by eating one kind of fruit every two to four days. Please go slowly. Fruits have a high natural sugar content and you don't want to reverse the progress you have made. Even if fruits are safe for you, limit them to one a day, and in a week or more, see if you can tolerate progressing to one per meal while on the program.

Don't be disappointed if you find you do not yet tolerate fruits. Many people find they cannot tolerate fruits with other foods, especially grains, because the combination sets up a fermentation reaction. In this case, only eat fruits alone, between meals, and have no other foods an hour before or afterward.

The Yeast Challenge

The yeast challenge also should be done only after you have become clear of all symptoms for at least two weeks.

You can challenge with small amounts of fresh breads containing only organic flour, salt, water, and yeast, including essene bread, or organic sprouted whole grain bread. Next you could challenge the vinegars like Bragg's, apple cider vinegar, or other vinegars. Never use distilled white vinegar.

If you have no reactions, you may want to add some yeast and fermented foods back into your diet. Please go slowly and if you show any adverse symptoms hold off adding these foods back for a while longer. If you can tolerate them, and only when you can eat anything for a limited time and do not trigger yeast symptoms, consider them as occasional treats only until you are sure you have "beaten the yeast."

Recipes

These recipes and menus were designed by the author of *Macro Mellow,* Shirley Gallinger, who for over two decades has also been an awesome friend and allergy assistant. We have provided basics to help folks start on their road to wellness by beginning an anti-Candida program. Use as many healthful, whole, and fresh ingredients as possible. For example, pan oils should not be the spray-on type, but good-quality cooking oil, like extra virgin olive oil and cold-pressed vegetable and nut oils. Avoid the grocery-store hydrogenated oils, margarines, and shortenings that are loaded with artery- and membrane-damaging trans fatty acids.

Lemon-Oil-Herb Vinaigrette

(3–4 servings)

5 tbsp virgin olive oil	1 tbsp freshly chopped herbs (any
2 tbsp fresh lemon juice	combination of parsley, chive,
¼ tsp sea salt or to taste	basil, tarragon, thyme)

Combine all ingredients in a glass jar and shake very well or blend in blender. Pour over salad greens and toss well. **Be creative:** Try cilantro and more unusual herbs as well.

Bragg's Lemon Dressing

Use Bragg's Liquid Amino Acids (unfermented and available in health food stores) alone or with the juice of a fresh lemon on salads and steamed vegetables.

Green Goddess Dressing

(Serves 4)

4 oz tofu (crumbled soft tofu)   ⅛ tsp white pepper
3 fresh spinach leaves   ¼ cup pure water
1 finely chopped scallion   1½ tbsp lemon or lime juice
1½ tbsp fresh basil   ½ cup oil of your choice
¼ tsp sea salt

Place all ingredients except for oil in blender and process until liquefied. With blender at low speed, slowly add oil in a steady stream until the dressing is thick and creamy. Cover and refrigerate until ready to serve. Will stay fresh for a week if refrigerated.

Fennel-Onion Salad

1 Whole Fennel
1 Onion (Vidalia or sweet red)
Pine Nuts (optional)

Grate fennel root and onion. Toss with lemon-oil vinaigrette or green goddess dressing. Sprinkle in pine nuts (optional). Serve cold or a room temperature.

Almond Milk

(Serves 4–6)

1 cup almonds   1 tbsp oil (almond oil if possible)
4 cups pure water   dash sea salt

Drop almonds into boiling water to cover. Boil for thirty seconds, remove from heat and let sit for three minutes. Drain and squeeze the skins from the almonds. Combine almonds with remaining ingredients in a blender and blend for two minutes.

Line a colander or strainer with two layers of cheesecloth and strain liquid. Squeeze out as much liquid as possible. Store in covered container in the refrigerator. Extra can be frozen.

The strained almond meal can be made into almond sprinkles by roasting gently on a cookie sheet until dry and golden. Delicious over cereals or salads. May lightly season with sea salt or Herbamare if desired.

This same recipe can be used with cashew and filberts. (Cashews do not have to be blanched in hot water since there are no skins and they are softer.)

Sesame Milk (Great for Cooking)

Yields 2½ cups

⅓ cup raw sesame seeds   2½ cup pure water, divided

Wash sesame seeds in cold water and drain well. Place in blender with ½ cup of water and blend on high speed for one minute. Add remaining water and blend again. Can be used immediately for cooking purposes or refrigerated for future use.

Better Butter (Better for Your Health)

1 stick (½ cup) unsalted butter at room temperature
½ cup pure flaxseed oil

With electric mixer, blend together until light and fluffy. Store in refrigerator in glass container. Will be spreadable when cold. Use as you would butter.

Ferment-Free Mayonnaise

Makes almost 2 cups

2 large free-range eggs at room
   temperature, preferably organic
2 tbsp fresh lemon juice
¼ tsp sea salt

¼ tsp dry mustard powder
1¼ cup cold-pressed oil (safflower
   or sunflower)

Be sure all items are at room temperature before preparing. Combine eggs, lemon juice, sea salt, and dry mustard powder in blender. Blend at high speed for one minute. Very slowly add oil in a thin stream while blending at high speed. Continue blending until the mixture becomes thick and creamy. Store in a glass container in the refrigerator.

Mystery Mayonnaise

Makes 1½–2 cups

¼ cup almonds, blanched
¼ cup pure water
2 tbsp fresh lemon juice
¼ tsp dry mustard

⅛ tsp turmeric
¼ tsp sea salt
1 to 1½ cup mild oil (almond or walnut are nice)

Place blanched almonds and water in blender and blend until a thick cream forms. If the blender refuses to move, add a few drops of water until the blade moves freely. Add seasonings and blend briefly. With the blender running slowly, add oil through the top opening until the mixture will not absorb any more oil. Place in a glass jar and refrigerate. Can be reblended if needed, before serving. May substitute cashews for almonds for an extra-rich taste. Will keep at least a week.

Tip: Mayonnaise can be thinned with any tolerated liquids and fresh herbs added to make a ranch-style dressing for salads.

Humus (Garbanzo or Chickpea Dip and Spread)

Serves 6

2 cups cooked garbanzo
   (chickpea) beans
   (well drained, save the liquid)
¼ cup cooking liquid
¼ cup tahini butter (optional)

2 tbsp olive oil
2 tbsp lemon juice
1 tsp minced garlic
½ tsp sea salt

Combine in food processor or blender cooked garbanzo beans, 2 tbsp of reserved cooking liquid, lemon juice, and olive oil. Blend until well mashed, adding more cooking liquid if needed. Blend in the tahini, garlic, and seasonings. Do not overblend. The texture should be creamy and rough at the same time. If using a blender, it may be necessary to process in several smaller batches. Cover and refrigerate until ready to serve. Serve with raw vegetables or yeast-free breads, biscuits, or crackers. The traditional dipper is pita bread, which does contain yeast; after you beat the yeast you will be able to use it.

Sauerkraut Dip

¼ cup mayonnaise

½–⅓ cup organic sauerkraut made with only sea salt and water

1 clove garlic, minced

¼ tsp of cumin (to taste)

Blend all (try a mini, handheld blender that is easy to clean; available in gourmet shops); serve with a mixture of attractively cut vegetables for dipping. Play with the proportions and add other herbs. Turmeric adds a nice yellow color. This should become one of your staples, since it is a wonderful way to make raw veggies more enticing and it provides a daily dose of healing garlic as well as sauerkraut. Although technically a ferment, it is generally well tolerated. Test yourself first by getting clear of symptoms on a more restricted diet, then add this in. If you stay clear of symptoms, it is OK for you. Some tolerate the sauerkraut better if it is rinsed before use.

Almond Dip

(Serves 6)

½ lb tofu, mashed

3 tbsp lemon juice

2 tbsp oil

⅛ tsp stevia (stevia to equal sweetness of 2 tsp sugar)

½ tsp sea salt or to taste

¼ cup roasted chopped almonds

Blend the first five ingredients in blender until smooth and creamy. Pour into a bowl and fold in the chopped almonds. Chill briefly before serving. Great with raw veggies or plain rice crackers.

By eliminating the tofu, lemon, and stevia, you have almond butter. You may want to thin with water.

Corn Muffins

12 servings (of one muffin)

1¼ cup whole-wheat flour

¾ cup yellow corn meal

4½ tsp baking powder (Rumford, aluminum-free from catalogs in resource section)

½ tsp sea salt

1 egg

⅔ cup water or nut milk

⅓ cup safflower or sunflower oil (or ganic and cold-pressed)

Combine dry ingredients in large mixing bowl. Blend egg, water or nut milk, and oil together. Combine liquid mixture with dry mixture and stir until just moistened. Don't overbeat. Divide mixture into twelve muffin cups. Bake at 425° F. for twenty to thirty minutes. Extra muffins freeze well.

Sweet Potato Muffins

12 Servings

1 cup whole-wheat pastry flour
1 cup unbleached white flour
½ tsp baking soda
½ tsp sea salt
2 tsp baking powder
  (Rumford aluminum-free)

½ tsp cinnamon
½ cup cooked, pureed sweet potatoes
⅓ cup oil
1 cup nut milk
½ cup chopped nuts (optional)

Preheat oven to 400° F and prepare muffin tin. Combine dry ingredients in a large mixing bowl and set aside. Combine cooked sweet potatoes with rest of liquid ingredients.

Chop nuts if using. Combine wet ingredients with dry ingredients and mix just enough to moisten. Add nuts if desired. Spoon into prepared muffin tins and bake for about twenty-five minutes or until done. Delicious served hot: the sweet potato gives the sweet flavor.

Note: If you have the basket-type juicer, you can substitute leftover carrot juice pulp for sweet potatoes. You may need to add liquid or a pinch of maple syrup, if tolerated, depending on the sweetness of the carrots.

Whole-Wheat Tortillas

A delicious flatbread with no yeast. Great with veggie or bean fillings and formed into a sandwich for lunch or a snack.

1 cup whole-wheat flour
1 cup unbleached, unbromated
  all-purpose flour
1 tsp sea salt

3 tbsp vegetable oil
½ cup warm water (or slightly more
  if needed)
whole-wheat flour as needed

Combine all ingredients in a large bowl to make a light-textured dough. Form into eight egg-sized balls, and place the balls in the bowl. Let stand for about twenty minutes.

Roll each ball of dough out on a lightly floured board to form a very thin circle, about ⅛ inch thick.

Lightly oil a griddle or large skillet and fry each tortilla over medium-low heat for a minute on one side, then a minute on the other. When the first side is done, the tortilla will begin to puff up. Turn it over, fry the other side. They will be slightly browned in spots, not all over. Serve warm. Will make eight large tortillas. Recipe may be doubled.

You can also often find wheat tortillas or corn tortillas in your health food store. Just be sure to check ingredients to be sure they do not contain yeast. Tortillas can add even more variety to your diet: cut into triangles for warm olive oil and fresh chopped-garlic dip or for sandwiches for work and travel.

Beef-Barley-Vegetable Soup

1 lb stew beef cut into small 1-inch pieces
⅓ cup whole barley

In a large pot, sauté the stew beef in olive oil on low-medium heat until well browned. Add barley and eight cups of water or your vegetable water saved from cooking. Simmer for approximately one hour or until beef and barley are tender.

Add:

1 cup finely sliced carrots	1 clove garlic
1 cup chopped celery	2 cups chopped fresh tomatoes
½ cup chopped onion	

Simmer just a few minutes until vegetables are tender, but before they lose their bright color. In fact, if you make a large amount, just add the veggies to the amount you will be serving immediately. You may add fresh vegetables to the soup before serving on another day. Season with salt and pepper and garnish each bowl with freshly chopped parsley. Leftovers can be frozen for another day.

Gingered Leek and Lentil Soup

(Serves 4–6)

½ lb lentils (about 2 cups)	1 tbsp minced garlic
8 cups of water or vegetable broth	1 tbsp minced fresh ginger root
2 tbsp olive oil	1 tsp Braggs' Liquid Amino Acids
2 cups chopped leeks	(not fermented, soy sauce flavor)

Wash lentils and add to the eight cups of hot vegetable broth. Let set for fifteen minutes. While soaking the lentils in the broth, sauté the leeks in oil for three to four minutes, until softened. (Do not brown.) Add garlic and ginger and sauté for two to three minutes longer. Combine with lentils and broth and simmer until lentils are tender but not mushy, about twenty-five minutes.

Remove from heat and stir in Braggs' Liquid Amino Acids seasoning sauce. Check for seasonings and serve hot. Leftovers reheat well.

Squash Soup

1 buttercup squash, seeded but not peeled
1 cup chicken broth (best if rendered from your own leftover organic chicken bones)

1 clove garlic, peeled and minced
5 leaves of chopped fresh basil
1 large sweet (Vidalia, if available) onion, finely chopped
1 tsp sea salt

Cook twenty minutes or until all veggies are soft, adding more water if need. Cool, blend, thin as needed with water, veggie or chicken broth, or nut milk. Reheat, serve with garnish of chopped scallions.

Cabbage-Carrot Slaw

(Serves 3–4)

¼ head of medium sized cabbage
2 carrots
4 finely sliced scallions
Sunflower seeds

¼ cup chopped parsley
Ferment-free mystery mayonnaise (as needed)

Grate cabbage and carrots into a large bowl, add sliced scallions and chopped parsley. Blend in mayonnaise. Check for seasonings and add sea salt and pepper if needed. Place in serving bowl and sprinkle sunflower, caraway, or sesame seeds over top.

Barley Nut Salad

(Serves 4–6)

1 cup uncooked whole barley
⅓ cup wheat berries
2⅔ cups pure water
½ cup fresh lemon juice
⅓ cup extra virgin olive oil
½ tsp sea salt

3 stalks of celery, finely chopped
2 carrots, finely chopped
1 sweet onion, finely chopped
½ to 1 cup minced fresh parsley or cilantro (optional)
½ cup roasted nuts (walnuts, almonds, or pecans)

Wash barley and wheat berries and combine with water in a large saucepan. Bring to boil. Reduce heat and simmer until all water is absorbed and the grains are tender, about 50 minutes.

Allow cooked grains to cool while preparing the vegetables and dressing. Wash and chop vegetables. Mince parsley, roast and chop nuts. Combine lemon juice, oil, and salt. Combine all ingredients and mix thoroughly. Check for seasonings and adjust if needed.

Refrigerate several hours before serving to blend flavors. Can be served on a bed of fresh salad greens.

Alaska Salmon Salad

The best canned salmon we've found comes from Seafood Direct (1-800-732-1836).

1 can salmon (If you order the chinook, it has those great edible bones, loaded with calcium)
mystery mayonnaise

chopped Vidalia or other onion and celery
ground black or white pepper to taste

Stuff mixture in half a peeled avocado or large celery stalks, place on a bed of Romaine lettuce, or use safe breads, which become even tastier when toasted.

Getting More Garlic

Since most of the thousands of species of yeasts are sensitive to the phytochemicals in garlic, let's look at some of the many ways to increase your daily intake of garlic.

1. Blend minced garlic into salad dressings.
2. Sauté garlic with oil and add to steamed veggies.
3. Make an olive oil dip for safe breads or veggies, adding ground herbs like oregano. Or use the sauerkraut dip with plenty of garlic for veggies.
4. Add a clove to carrot juice, but limit fresh veggie juice to one half to three quarters cup a day until symptoms improve and you can evaluate the effect of larger amounts.
5. Use odorless garlics. Kyolic aged garlic capsules, two capsules three to four times a day plus Garlitrin 4000 or Garlinase 4000 once a day are excellent sources. The reason I use two different types is that different manufacturing processes result in different yeast-killing phytochemicals. (See Resource Guide.)

How to Get More Healing Veggies into the Diet

The Candida diet can be just the beginning of a healthier "you"; enjoy the adventure. But you can speed things up by getting three to four veggies per meal. Being creative gets you healthier quicker:

1. Become a creative cut-up. Cut veggies in unusual ways and into smaller pieces to enhance flavor, then store in iced water with sea salt.
2. Use veggie dips—humus, almond, avocado, sauerkraut—to enhance appeal.
3. Experiment with yogurt and herbs, flavored mayonnaise, tofu, squash, pâté (minced meats with better butter, mayo, etc.).

Beyond the Diet

For all products recommended, see Resource Guide for suppliers.

Overcoming Cravings

Don't let hunger sabotage your progress. It may mean that you are fat starved, in which case have more oils and fats, nuts and nut butters. A great way of improving your fatty acid status with the three most commonly deficient fatty acids is with a daily teaspoonful of Carlson's Cod Liver Oil (contains DHA and EPA) or if you need your fish oil in capsules, take three capsules of Tyler's Eskimo-3 daily, for both are of excellent quality and cover the most commonly low omega-3 oil deficiencies that trigger cravings, lower reisistance to Candida, and cause many, including gut, symptoms. In addition, you may want to take either three capsules of Efamol's Evening Primrose Oil one to two times a day or Thorne's Black Current Oil, two to three caps twice a day to cover the most commonly deficient omega-6 oil.

Because deficiencies in omega-3 levels are more common, correct your omega-3 intake first. If you don't notice any improvement in even a subtle symptom within two months, switch to omega-6, or better yet, have your levels measured. (See Chapter 7.) Usually when correcting an essential fatty acid deficiency, there are a number of subtle improvements, like softer skin, loss of dermatitis, better hair texture, or happier moods. Once you have corrected your fatty acid deficiencies, you will have fewer cravings as well. If your symptoms worsen, back off and take only one oil at a time to determine which you may *not* need.

Sweets to Cheat With

Cravings for sweets, although a classic symptom of Candida overgrowth, usually dissipate within a week or two of starting the program. If they persist, you may need to "cheat": You could make tofu turtles and other more wholesome "sweets" (in *Macro Mellow*), or use more nut butters, perhaps over a frozen banana or blended and frozen with a banana as a treat that resembles ice cream. But remember, the most common cause of persistent cravings for sweets is undetected mineral deficiencies. And the most common mineral deficiencies that trigger hypoglycemia are chromium, manganese, magnesium, and vanadium. Get a mineral panel (described in Chapter 7) drawn or start the regimen outlined in the preceding chapter.

"What If I Just Ignore This 'Harmless' Yeast?"

If the thought has crossed your mind, it suggests you just don't have time to fit the program into your life right now. But buck up. Chances are you don't need to do even a fourth of what I've presented here. For many folks, getting rid of yeasts and gaining a new lease on life is as easy as doing the diet, probiotics, a garlic derivative and Paragard for four to eight weeks. (More about this in Chapter 5.) Before the four to eight weeks are up, these people are feeling better than they have in years as symptoms melt away and friends ask them what they are doing to look and feel so great. Some can improve with even less effort. No one knows how severe your case is. But one thing is clear: untreated Candida overgrowth is a major cause of chronic gut symptoms. In addition to healing the gut, most folks also lose a half dozen or more other symptoms that they never thought were related.

Leaving yeast overgrowth untreated invites an avalanche of symptoms from the leaky gut that can lead to nutritional deficiencies, chemical sensitivity, food allergy, or autoimmune disease, chronic fatigue, and more. The Candida toxin, acetaldehyde, can cause brain fog (dizziness or inability to concentrate), depression, bizarre body aches like fibromyalgia, and more.

Start with a Cleaner Gut and Fewer Organisms

Nature's Pure Body Purification Program (Pure Body Institute). There are two bottles in this package. Take one to four tablets of the colon-cleansing bottle portion and three to eight tablets of the herbal body purification portion, one to three times a day for two to fifteen days. You can use it for one to two months if you choose. By cleansing the gut and improving the transit time, this will lessen die-off, cravings, gut symptoms, and prepare a welcome bed for probiotics, making it easier for the Candida-killers to do their work.

Probiotics

You must put some healthy "good" bugs back in the intestine so that when your yeast program is done, the yeasts do not just regrow, returning you to the ill health you've recovered from. Probiotics, the best way to get healthful competing bugs, also have other beneficial effects contributing to a healthy gut and immune system, and they lower cholesterol, improve your resistance to infections, and make gut cells less prone to cancer.

You can measure if you have sufficient levels of the two most common probiotics, or beneficial bacteria, *Lactobacillus acidophilus* and *Bifidus*, in the intestines, when you culture the stool (comprehensive digestive stool assay [CDSA]—as described in Chapter 6).

You can start building your probiotic levels with powder or capsule form. Klaire Laboratory's VitalPlex, one teaspoon in water twice a day, or Kyodophilus, Enterogenic Concentrate, Natrens or DDS acidophilus are among the many to choose from; one to two capsules or one-half to one teaspoon should be taken twice a day. Most forms work best before or between meals, so that the gastric juices do not kill them.

Always test your probiotics by taking a double or triple dose once. If it causes tremendous gas for a few hours, the organisms are alive and growing well in your gut. Then cut back to a dose that does not cause gas. If your probiotic is dead, or your stomach acid is killing them before they get to the small intestine where they live, you are wasting your money and should change brands. Although I discuss probiotics in more detail in Chapter 4, the brief review given here will get you started.

When you are better, remember that the probiotics are the last thing to stop in the program, outside of the diet. That is because many of the yeast-fighters also kill some of the good bugs. So you need to be sure to continue the probiotics about a month beyond your last yeast-fighter. High levels of the good bugs discourage yeasts from ever showing up again. Also, even though all the reports say that fructo-oligosaccharides (FOS) are safe for folks fighting Candida, I have found a significant number of folks who tell me that FOS definitely makes their Candida symptoms worse. So watch out for this rare event.

Nonprescription Yeast Fighters

There are many over-the-counter yeast fighters that can help with the battle. You can choose from among them, or see which ones your particular type of yeast is most sensitive to. If you had your stool cultured, most likely the lab included in the doctor's report a sensitivity test to determine which remedies would work best to kill your type of yeast, or you can experiment on your own.

Since many of these products work by different mechanisms against yeast, you may want to use several brands in combination. You do not need all brands, and there are many others if these fail. Some folks can reverse symptoms easily by following the beat-the-yeast diet and by taking one or two of the nonprescription yeast fighters for one to four months, as listed below. Whatever yeast fighter you use, be sure to continue taking your probiotics for two to four weeks afterward to ensure the growth of good bugs.

Paragard (Tyler), two to three capsules, three times a day between meals.
> Description of contents and actions of this herbal bug fighter can be found in Chapter 4.

Garlinase or Garlitrin 4000 (Enzymatic Therapy), once a day.
> Source of garlic phytochemicals that kill yeast.

Kyolic (Wakunaga), two capsules twice a day.
> Source of different garlic phytochemicals that kill yeast.

AquaPhase A (30C homeopathic), two tablespoons in four tablespoons water daily on an empty stomach.
> Homeopathic anti-Candida remedy.

WaterOz Silver Mineral Water (WaterOz), one teaspoon in water, one to two times a day.
> Easily assimilated low-dose form of silver which is antibacterial, antifungal, and antiprotozoal.

Aloe Vera Drink (Klaire Labs, Carlson Labs, Aloe Products of North America), two to three ounces, one to two times a day.
> Juice of succulent or cactus that has proven healing properties on contact.

Aloe Gel Caps (Carlson), use one to four every two to five hours as need.
> For the power of an entire cup of aloe juice concentrated into a potent capsule.

Kapricidin-A (Ecologic Formulas) contains 325 milligrams caprylic acid, one to six capsules two to three times a day with meals. Always start at the lowest dose and advance slowly every few days. It is always better to tolerate a small amount of healing nutrients than get an even more irritated stomach from too many. There is no prize for getting to the top recommended dose with speed. In fact many do very well with never achieving the top doses of anything. And if for any reason you do not tolerate any of these, you still have lots of options. Many folks only take 2-3 products to rid themselves of Candida.

A fatty acid with anti-Candida properties.

ParaMicrocidin (Purity Research/ARG) is citrus seed extract, 250 milligrams, one to two capsules, two to three times a day. Alternatively, PCN-200 (Bio-Tech) is 200 milligrams or Paracan-Myc (Ecologic Formulas) is 200 milligrams of seed and pulp bioflavonoid polyphenols, of which you may take two to six capsules with meals.

Phytochemical from citrus seeds that have Anti-Candida properties.

Oil of Oregano drops (North American Herb & Spice or ARG), two to six drops under the tongue or in water, two to four times a day, or as Oregamax capsules. The phytochemicals of oregano are also antibacterial, antifungal, and antiprotozoal.

On the other hand, because they also can kill the beneficial bugs, you need to reestablish the good bugs (see probiotics described in this and following chapters after treating with Oil of Oregano (Zaika).

Biocidin (BioBotanical), four to six drops in water three times a day with meals or one to four tablets with meals.

A proprietary compound of herbs with antibacterial and anti-Candida properties.

Undecyn (Thorne), one to three capsules three times a day. A fatty acid derived from the castor bean plant, it is six times more effective than caprylic acid. The calcium salt of undecyn is combined with betaine to promote utilization; it also has yeast-fighting grapefruit seed extract and toxin-sponging bentonite.

Dioxychlor DC3 (American Biologics), five to twenty drops one to three times a day in water or under the tongue.

A chlorinated oxygen product that has anti-Candida properties.

Paracidin (Ecologic Formulas), one to three capsules an hour before meals. Contains activated charcoal to absorb Candida toxins for folks having trouble tolerating anything. In addition it has tannic acid which discourages Candida growth, and iodine, a mineral used by medicine before antibiotics were available to kill unwanted bugs in the gut.

Tanalbit (N.E.E.D.S.), follow package directions.

Restore lost minerals with Biomin II (Thorne) for a month after, as this tannic acid product can kill yeast, but also inhibits mineral absorption.

Lactoferrin (Ecologic Formula), one to four capsules (100 milligrams) twice daily between meals. A specialized iron-binding protein with anti-

Candida properties endemic to mother's milk. As an adjunct to Lactoferrin, some folks benefit even more with the addition of Nutricillin (Ecologic Formulas), at the same dosage. In addition to 60 milligrams more Lactoferrin, Nutricillin contains olive leaf extract (50 mg) and colostrum (150 mg), both well-studied for their own antimicrobial actions.

Package Programs

Or if you prefer, there are package programs I put together for patients using the products designed by several fine companies. (Addresses, phone numbers, and alternate suppliers in Resource Guide). The doses and combinations are mine, not the companies', and many of the products have unusually formulated items that are especially helpful for certain individuals who have tried all other nonprescription possibilities. Each package includes one or more items to kill Candida, restore beneficial flora, improve bowel cleansing, support the immune system, or enhance healing of the lining of the entire gastrointestinal tract. You do not necessarily have to use all the products in one list, although they are synergistic.

Wakunaga Program

Kyolic, two twice a day
Kyo-Green, one to three heaping teaspoons in eight ounces water two to
    eight times a day, anytime
Kyo-Dophilus, one to two capsules twice a day with food

(Free samples of all three available from 1-800-825-7888)

Tyler Program

Paragard, two to three capsules three times a day between meals
Enterogenic Concentrate, one to two teaspoons one to two times a day,
    before or between meals
Fiber Formula, one to two capsules with large glasses of water, one to
    two times a day (cut back if more than three stools a day or too loose)
Candida Complex, two to four with meals

PhytoPharmica (Enzymatic Therapy) Program

Garlitrin 4000, one to two a day
ZymeDophilus, one capsule three times a day with meals

FiberPlus, two to six capsules a day with one to two large glasses of
   water
Candimyacin, one to two between meals, two to three times a day

Thorne Program

Citricidin, one to four capsules three to four times a day, anytime
Undecyn, two to three capsules three times a day
Lactobacillus sporogenes, one capsule two to three times a day
Herbal Bulk, one to two teaspoons in large glass of water one to three
   times a day

Pure Encapsulations Program

A.C. Formula, one to two capsules before meals
Lactobacillus sporogenes, one to three capsules between meals
Garlic 100:1, one to two capsules a day with meals

Jarrow Program

Jarrow-Dophilus, one to two capsules one to two times a day, one half to
   one hour before eating
Yaeyama Chlorella, powder or capsules, follow package directions
Flax Fiber, one to two tablespoons in two large glasses of water

Support Nutrient Program

If you are still unable to conquer Candida, see Chapter 6. You may need
to heal a leaky gut first or to include the diagnostic diet to uncover hidden
food allergies, or eradicate other bugs before you are strong enough to
eliminate Candida.

Prescription Yeast Fighters

If Candida is too strongly entrenched in the gut to be eradicated with
nonprescription yeast fighters, it may be time for prescription varieties.
There are two categories: (1) those that are not absorbed but kill the yeast
from inside the gut (Nystatin pure powder), and (2) systemic yeast fighters,
which are absorbed and go to every cell in the body. These penetrate the gut
wall to kill Candida's mycelial fingers that reach inside the gut wall.

Nystatin

Nystatin is a prescription antifungal powder that most but not all yeasts are sensitive to. It is quite safe (although its taste does take getting used to) and is not absorbed into the system; it merely glides through the gut killing yeast on its way. One teaspoon three times a day is the top dose you can aim for. If you suspect severe sensitivity to Candida or severe die-off, begin with dot doses on the end of a toothpick and gradually increase to taking a full teaspoon as your symptoms allow. If you suspect a severe sensitivity, you should also do periodic colon cleanses (every six to eight weeks) and daily detoxification enemas as described in Chapter 6.

Nizoral, Difulcan, Sporonox

Once fungal overgrowth has been confirmed by stool culture, you will need a prescribed antifungal that goes into the bloodstream, such as Nizoral® (ketaconazole), Diflucan® (fluconazole), or Sporonox® (itraconazole). Unlike Nystatin, which just goes in the gut and out with the stool, these antifungals go inside the gut lumen or canal and then into the bloodstream, penetrating the gut wall (i.e., the lining of the entire GI tract). This is important because it is in the gut wall that Candida's fungal mycelia act like fingers as they avidly reach in between gut wall cells and cling for life. Again, sensitivity tests will guide physicians as to which antifungal is most likely to do the best job.

The Candida Program Reviewed

Complete all the steps as given below only if you need to. If you start feeling better at any step along the way, then stop there until all symptoms vanish completely.

1. Diagnose Candida with a 7-Day Candida Culture.
2. Purge intestines with laxative to reduce or avoid die-off.
3. Begin the yeast-free, sugar-free, ferment-free diet and do not add back foods until you are free of symptoms.
4. Begin the probiotic regimen.
5. Begin taking the nonprescription antifungals. When in doubt, the herbal preparations Paragard, Kyolic, and Garlitrin 4000 are a good start.
6. Evaluate other combinations or some of the package programs (taking each one for at least a month before switching to another).
7. Look at what may be missing from your total load that inhibits your

body from fighting off a yeast like Candida—or any other bug for that matter.

8. See your physician for a prescription for Nystatin, slowly working up to top dose from the dot dose as previously described. Your physician will probably insist on at least a 7-Day Candida Culture (see Chapter 6) to confirm the diagnosis. The only drawback, as you will read later, is that the test misses in five to ten precent of cases and only a therapeutic trial (which is harmless) will tell if Candida is the cause of your symptoms.

"What If I'm Not Better?"

1. Be sure you have been correctly diagnosed. (See Chapter 7.)
2. The most common reason for failure is eating foods that are not on the diet. If you need more details on the diet, read *The E. I. Syndrome.*
3. You may need a prescription from your doctor for Nystatin, Nizoral, Diflucan, or other yeast fighters.
4. Get further diagnostic tests to see if you have another condition that needs healing before you can effectively kill off the yeast. Common roadblocks include undiagnosed mineral, fatty acid, or vitamin deficiencies; heavy metal toxicities; hypoglycemia; leaky gut; overloaded total load; damaged detoxification system; among others. These are described in Chapter 7 and in more detail in my book *Depression Cured At Last!*
5. Do a daily detoxification enema (Chapter 6) and/or periodic body purification protocol (Chapter 5) every six to twelve weeks. This step is optional if you do not have severe or particularly resistant Candida.
6. **Remember:** Candida overgrowth is curable. It is only a question of finding out why you are still so vulnerable, which I will discuss in subsequent chapters.

Staying Well

Diet, food combining, chewing, probiotics, whey, digestive enzymes, and many other adjuncts can keep the bowel functioning well once you have relieved your symptoms.

The Whey of Healing

"Little Miss Muffet, sat on a tuffet, eating her curds and whey." Why? Because she knew something that many people have forgotten: Whey is a great way to alkalinize the bowel.

Who needs to alkalinize bowel? Anyone with foul-smelling intestinal gas, lots of gas and bloating and indigestion, or who cannot keep the good bugs in the gut for very long. For when the bowel gets too acidic from diets high in meat, sweets and sodas, or processed foods, it cannot support the growth of the good bacteria that keep the gut's immune system healthy. These folks endlessly take probiotics in an attempt to restore the flora to the gut, but it just dies off again because of the unfriendly acidic background.

During the cheese-making process, enzymes are added to milk to curdle it, resulting in curds of cheese and the liquid whey, which has been used for centuries as a healthful drink. Now you don't have to make your own cheese in order to benefit from the healing whey.

To heal your intestines, try taking one to three tablespoons of whey a day. It can be mixed in cereal or cooking (for instance, anywhere you would add milk, such as in a white sauce) and is generally safe for lactose-intolerant folks who can eat yogurt. You can order whey from Wakunaga of America (1-800-825-7888); they will also send you a free sample each of Kyolic, a garlic supplement for killing intestinal yeast overgrowth, and Kyo-Dophilus, the probiotic of *Lactobacillus acidophilus.* Once you have killed the undesirable and restored the good organisms, if you have an alkaline bowel, it should stay healthy. Other great sources include Thorne and Jarrow.

In a Nutshell

Although Candida, a normally harmless yeast, is the most common infection that causes gut symptoms, seldom do doctors look for it. As we've seen, Candida can also cause myriad other body symptoms.

A healthy body, not a powerful drug, can overcome Candida. As countless people have told me over a quarter of a century, following the Candida program is one of the best things they ever did for their gut, as well as for their overall physical and mental health and energy. The day you start to beat the yeast may well be the beginning of the first feelings of total health you have ever known!

CHAPTER 4

Bugs: The Good, the Bad, and the Deadly

Helicobacter pylori: The Common Bug That Causes Ulcers and Stomach Cancer

Who would believe a common bacterium that contaminates a multitude of foods and city water supplies in the United States can cause ulcers? And if the presence of this bacterium is not diagnosed and treated, that it can go on to cause stomach cancer? Such was the frustration of an Australian doctor, Barry Marshall, when he tried to interest the drug-driven medical profession in his important findings. They just did not want to believe them and ignored him for over a decade. But what a paradigm shift he has caused since. In the case of some early stomach cancers, we now know that by diagnosing and treating *Helicobacter pylori* (also known as *Campylobacter pylori*) we can cause the cancer to regress and disappear! This is the first time in the history of medicine that treating an infectious agent with an antibiotic has made a cancer disappear.

It is important for you to be aware of *H. pylori* because it can cause or mimic upset stomach, acid indigestion, gastritis, dyspepsia, and ulcers. Unrecognized, of course, it can go on to cause cancer of the stomach (Forman, Parsonnet, Uemura, Gross). In one study, *H. pylori* was the cause of stomach cancer in 63 percent of the patients; it was also discovered that 94 percent had made antibodies to the bug for thirteen years prior to the cancer when saved blood was reexamined (Nomura). Why is it important to know this? The answer is simple: Traditional medicine commonly ignores causes by suppressing symptoms with medication.

H. pylori Is Everywhere

Studies have shown that more than one in three folks with gastric symptoms harbors *H. pylori* and that it is a common contaminant of foods and water supplies. Needless to say, its role in causing ulcers and, when untreated, the cancer risk it poses, combined with its ease of treatment, make it imperative to look for this bacterium as one treatable cause of any upper-abdominal symptoms.

Indeed, researchers have found in some populations that they studied for *H. pylori,* as much as 60 percent of them had it (Eurogast Study Group). The bacterium has even been found in household cats. In light of such data, think for a moment of millions of bottles of antacids and H2-blockers on drugstore and supermarket shelves waiting to be carried home by those one in three folks who really ought to be resolving the cause of their upset and thereby preventing future stomach cancer as well. These uninformed folks are actually taking medications that are like fertilizer to *H. pylori*—by reducing stomach acid, they allow *H. pylori* to flourish!

This bug is so common that, in one study (Boren), more than 60 percent of those over sixty years of age had *H. pylori* residing in their stomachs. In another study, 68 percent of the spouses of people with *H. pylori* also had the infection (Riccardi). The problem is that some folks can have asymptomatic infection or very mild, intermittent symptoms. In others, the bug can cause insidious, painless rotting away of the stomach lining (called gastric atrophy or atrophic gastritis), leading to such serious malabsorption of minerals and other nutrients as to contribute to problems like osteoporosis, hypertension, angina, Parkinson's disease, Tourette's syndrome, Alzheimer's disease, schizophrenia, depression, premature aging, senility, and cancer.

A Cause of Slow, Mysterious Decline and Death

What's a little acid indigestion? How serious could it be? Well, it just could be the very first sign that you have of *H. pylori* infection. So if you have pain in the epigastrium, the upper abdomen, just below the breastbone, or in the pit of your stomach and do not have an ulcer, hiatus hernia, or cancer that can be seen on an X ray, then your condition is certain. You have nonulcer dyspepsia (NUD), or gastritis, or epigastritis, or functional dyspepsia. They all mean pretty much the same thing. It all boils down to "We haven't the foggiest notion of why your upper stomach hurts; but we know it is not yet an ulcer or cancer."

But I'll tell you that anyone who diagnoses one of these conditions without making sure you do not have *H. pylori* infection should be fired if he or she merely tries to prescribe a drug for you. It is abundantly clear now that vast sums of money and many lives can be saved by screening for *H. pylori* whenever there is a gastric problem (Fendrick, Hood).

If untreated or enhanced by common drug therapy, *H. pylori* can do the same thing to the stomach lining that gluten does to the lining of the small intestine of those with celiac disease. It denudes the surface and renders it useless. When this happens to the stomach lining, atrophic gastritis results, which can lead to a slow, painful death by multiple diseases.

With deficient or no acid secretion in the stomach, you cannot fight off the many bacteria, fungi, and parasites that you ingest in a day. Nor can you digest your foods completely, or absorb nutrients like calcium, iron, folic acid, or B_6 and B_{12}. Certainly, without these nutrients, it is tough to heal any gut problem, much less to increase your resistance to further invasion. These same deficiencies can then precipitate an avalanche of undiagnosable symptoms from angina to insanity. Simply, with a defective stomach lining, there is not enough mucus to protect the stomach, making it vulnerable to infection, malabsorption, ulcers, or cancer.

As you slowly become depleted of nutrients, your symptoms will rise in number and severity. If you are an older individual, people may just chalk it up to your so-called age-related decline. In time, when enough of the gastric mucosa has died or atrophied, you won't even feel the pain that normally accompanies symptoms. It then becomes even more unlikely that a physician will look for *H. pylori* when larger problems, such as cardiomyopathy, congestive heart failure, or life-threatening cardiac arrhythmia—all from your mineral deficiencies—loom.

Gastric atrophy can also affect you in other ways. From the shutting off of the production of intrinsic factor in gastric parietal cells, which prohibits the absorption of vitamin B_{12}, you may encounter numbness, paralysis, painful neuropathy, depression, or even schizophrenia. In addition, gastric atrophy can cause a state of chronic indigestion that may arise as food lingers in a stomach beset by destroyed stomach cells that can no longer secrete pepsinogen or acid.

With more than 30 percent of folks over sixty years of age suffering from gastric atrophy, we now recognize it as a major cause of premature aging, that downhill deterioration we witness in aging friends and colleagues. How much of it is caused by *H. pylori* is anyone's guess. But if 60 percent of folks over sixty have *H. pylori,* it is most likely a principal cause of accelerated aging, along with its secondary form, gastric atrophy.

In children, an *H. pylori* infection can cause recurring abdominal pain, but will not show up on X rays. Like any other disease, you have to have a good suspicion to order the correct test. Rarely does the answer fall into your lap.

H. pylori's helical shape allows it to burrow in a corkscrew fashion into the protective mucous layer to infect one tiny part of the stomach, causing an ulcer. The good news (if you have a physician who looks for it) is that 70 to 92 percent of folks with duodenal or gastric ulcers have *H. pylori* found at the scene (Jancin). Symptoms can include nausea or vomiting. Should you notice a substance in the vomitus that looks like coffee grounds, it's usually old blood. Another sign of blood is dark or tarry stools. With either of these signs, be certain to find an excellent gastroenterologist. Don't be afraid to test his or her knowledge and ask how he or she would treat you. If he or she wants to scope and prescribe drugs without looking at your *H. pylori* status, find another gastroenterologist whose knowledge base is wider and who understands damage done by *H. pylori*.

How the Sick Get Sicker, Quicker, with Approved Drugs

H. pylori doesn't like the acidic environment of the stomach any better than other bugs do. But it does something unique to protect itself: It secretes the enzyme urease, which acts upon uric acid, generating its own ammonia and bicarbonate that neutralize the acidity around it. (This can cause one's breath to smell like ammonia, an important clue that should not be ignored.) By making an alkaline-protective shield about itself, it can continue to nibble away at the gut cells it so tenaciously clings to.

If you are ahead of me, you already appreciate how taking an antacid or an H2-blocker like Tagamet or Zantac actually feeds this bug (Kuipers). Again, it's like throwing gasoline on a fire. By taking nonprescription drugs to turn off any last bit of acid the stomach may secrete in its attempt to kill the *H. pylori,* you will give the bug a boost while kicking the host (you) in the butt.

If your doctor prescribes Prilosec, then you're in for worse trouble yet (Logan). But since drugs like Prilosec calm the stomach, no one realizes that the drug itself is feeding a bug that can cause cancer or gastric atrophy. Again, studies confirm that *H. pylori* antibodies have been present in folks years before they finally were diagnosed with cancer (Munoz). So all the while they were busy trying to medicate symptoms, their physicians were missing a golden opportunity to practice real medicine.

Fortunately, once *H. pylori* has been detected and eradicated, the atrophied gastric mucosa can heal (Borody, Kieper 1995), provided that the doctor also assessed and corrected the nutrient deficiencies that accompany the condition. Not only do high intakes of whole foods, primarily fruits and vegetables, and antioxidants decrease your risk for *H. pylori* infection, (Hwang), they are even more essential if you have to reverse any damage done by the infection. And not only can treatment cure an ulcer, but it can also reverse or cure gastric cancer (De Koster, Bayerdorffer, Wotherspoon).

Besides drugs meant to mask symptoms, what else can fuel the fires of *H. pylori?* Include here the foods that have been known to increase your chances for stomach cancer: alcohol, highly salted and pickled foods, fermented and smoked foods, and nitrites as found in hot dogs, bacon, and other preserved deli meats (Hwang). Add on the nonsteroidal anti-inflammatory drugs (NSAIDs), smoking, and diets high in processed foods. Stress also plays a role here. By putting your body into the sympathetic fight-or-flight response too much of the time, you can shut down the stomach's digestive acids entirely or in part.

Yes, *H. pylori* is a threat, and not only for stomach problems. Indeed, never before in the history of medicine have we uncovered a bacterium that can cause stomach cancer. Reversing or curing the cancer by eradicating the bug is even more shattering to traditional medical beliefs (De Koster). But *H. pylori's* impact on our defenses doesn't stop there. This sneaky bug can dwell anonymously in the gut for years while it silently damages our tumor suppressor genes (Calvert). In addition, it can suppress the immune system by altering one of its chief guardian cells, the monocyte (Knipp). It has even triggered some cases of rosacea, an adult acnelike condition that causes a ruddy nose and cheeks (Baker), which medicine in true form treats with constant doses of antibiotics (that cause Candida overgrowth) rather than finding a curable cause.

Treatment of *H. pylori:* The Drugstore Cure That Is Ignored

Currently, medical treatment for *H. pylori* infection involves a triple therapy of either three antibiotics or two antibiotics and—you guessed it—Prilosec. If the stomach burns, then shut off the acid-making mechanism. Right? Never mind that Prilosec increases your vulnerability to the bug and actually helps it dig into your mucosa and destroy the stomach lining more easily. When the symptom has vanished, the patient believes the doctor has done his or her job.

As you might now suspect, anyone who has had this bug in the stomach for who knows how long suffers from lowered immunity. Chances are there is more than just the *H. pylori* infection causing symptoms as well. It should come as no surprise then that treatment with antibiotics and Prilosec only improved the symptoms in 27 percent of patients (McColl). That is not the kind of treatment success I want; in fact, I'd call that a failure.

Medicine has not yet caught on to the concept of total load, meaning that usually more than one thing is wrong. Doctors do not usually look for hidden vitamin and mineral deficiencies, for example, that routinely accompany gastric symptoms of long duration. Nor do they look for Candida, hidden food allergies, or any of the myriad other proven causes of GI symptoms.

Sometimes included in the triple antibiotic regimen is metronidazole (known by its popular brand name Flagyl). This drug has so many side effects that some folks just can't tolerate it. They may feel like they have a serious case of the flu and ache all over, or, because it knocks out one of the main first-line enzymes for detoxifying everyday chemicals, become suddenly more sensitive to chemicals that never bothered them before. For example, they may not be able to think clearly in certain work or home areas just because of a new carpet, paint, or an aerosol cleanser.

Metronidazole converts to a mimic of vitamin B_1 (thiamin), thus effectively throwing a monkey wrench in thiamine pyrophosphokinase, an enzyme needed for thiamine use. The result is bizarre neurological (nerve and brain) symptoms that few doctors can diagnose (Alston). Instead of metronidazole, use Allithiamine (Ecologic Formulas) which is explained in Chapter 3.

There are many nasty side effects with the triple antibiotic therapy, and the worst involves Candida: it can secondarily provoke a very intense Candida infection. Be that as it many, doctors still commonly prescribe and recommend the H2-blockers and Prilosec, despite the fact that they are counterproductive in the long run and encourage *H. pylori's* transformation into a cancer-causing bug (Henschel). Prilosec, in addition to adding considerable expense to the program, can actually increase your chances of getting *H. pylori* tenfold—if you did not yet have it.

Fortunately, there is a simple and inexpensive remedy that has a high rate of cure and is available in every drugstore. But because it is cheap, readily available, and nonprescription, there is very little research devoted to it, although many antibiotic studies include it with their drugs because researchers know it increases cure rates (Noach, Henschel).

Bismuth subsalicylate, better known as Pepto-Bismol, is the remedy I'm speaking of. Two caplets four times a day, taken with meals and before bed, is best. Be aware that all the forms contain aluminum, and the tablet form contains saccharin—so use sparingly. In most cases, a two-week regimen will be sufficient.

Don't panic when you look in the morning mirror either. All forms of Pepto-Bismol are capable of giving you a black tongue, as well as black stools. Black stools can also be a sign of old blood from an actively bleeding site in the gut. Be absolutely sure that you can turn on and off the black stool by taking or not taking Pepto-Bismol. If you have black stools without taking Pepto-Bismol, see your doctor and find the cause immediately.

Alternatives to Pepto-Bismol include (1) a nonprescription supplement containing bismuth as well as deglycyrrhized licorice (DGL), which as you will learn is one of the best remedies for healing indigestion, ulcers, and gastritis. Take two to three Formula SF734 (Thorne) four times a day for four to eight weeks, or (2) Gastromet (Ecologic Formulas), which also contains a healing amount of DGL (250 mg) and other optimizing ingredients like vitamin U (isolated from cabbage juice and known to heal ulcers) and chlorophyll, same dose. A companion to either of these is Helicoactrin (Ecologic Formulas) with high sulfate mucin needed to heal a badly invaded and damaged gut, accompanied by many other aids, same dose.

Should you wish to assess the success of your therapy, then all you need is a simple blood test. When *H. pylori* attacks the stomach, the body defends itself by making antibodies to the bug. The longer the body tries to fight the infection, the higher the level, or titer, of antibodies. Conversely, as the bug dies off and the body no longer has to work so hard at defending itself, the blood antibody titer goes down. Your antibody level thus can tell you whether an infection is old or current, and whether your therapy is successful or not.

If the Pepto-Bismol cure does not suffice, I would still not recommend the medical alternative: that heavy dose of triple antibiotics now in vogue and constantly changing. The reason is simple: You would be a lot better off finding out why you are so unhealthy that the nonprescription approach does not work. After all, it is the integrity of your system that determines the success of a treatment program, not the virulence of the bug.

What can you do to make yourself more resistant and to boost your immune system? Lots of things. First, be sure you are eating whole foods. In fact, the more raw fruits and vegetables you eat, the better. In raw fruits and vegetables the natural enzymes, antioxidant vitamins, minerals, and detox phytochemicals are at their peak. In the beginning, if your gut does not tolerate them raw, lightly steam your fruits and vegetables. Fresh (meaning you juice it yourself) organic carrot juice with a slice or two or organic beet or cabbage, as it bathes the ulcer or gastric erosion in antioxidants, is healing for the stomach if consumed two to five times a day.

DGL Protocol: The Nonprescription Stomach Healer

If you never used DGL for stomach disorders, you've missed out on a centuries-old, nonprescription, nontoxic therapy proven to heal ulcers and gastritis. To begin with, DGL has cut the rate of gastritis caused by aspirin in half (Dehpour). So why don't rheumatologists recommend it for patients for whom they prescribe a lifetime of gastritis-causing NSAIDs? NSAIDs (nonsteroidal anti-inflammatory drugs like Motrin, Advil, and Aleve) are a major cause of gastritis. Instead, they prescribe additional drugs like H2-

blockers (Tagamet, Zantac), Prilosec, Cytotec or Sucralfate that can be as much as eight times more expensive, cause side effects and are guaranteed to eventually damage your health.

On the other hand, since DGL speeds healing, and has a long history of doing so, it should be an essential part of all drug programs for the stomach. For over 35 years, major medical journals have published research proving its effectiveness to be superior, even to the currently prescribed stomach medications (Doll, Lewis, Horwich, Morgan, Kassir, Turpie). For example, fewer patients experienced relapse or recurrence of ulcers when on DGL as compared to Tagamet, or antacids (Kassir), or Zantac (Glick). One reason DGL can outperform prescription drugs is that it makes stomach cells produce more of their protective and healing mucus (Baker, Tarnawski, Van Marle)—a feat no medication can match.

DGL also improves the immunity of the stomach cells through enhancing the production of secretin (Takeuchi), which no medication can match as well. This effect is so powerful that it enhances the killing of the virus that causes cold sores or aphthous ulcers (Das), protects liver cells from dying from hepatitis (Yoshikawa), and inhibits other virus growth (Pompei), even HIV, the AIDS virus (Ito). If that were not superlative potency with protection and no bad side effects rolled into one, it has many other uses, from stopping cholesterol from forming inside arteries (Fuhrman) to being an antiarthritis aid (Tangri).

DGL does the opposite of drugs. Rather than turn off normal function, it promotes it. Increasing the production of healing mucus and revving up the immune system of stomach cells is only part of its benefits. Because of its anti-inflammatory and antioxidant properties, DGL stimulates many avenues simultaneously that promote resistance to damage and speed up healing if damage has occurred.

The rate of recurrence of ulcers within a year now stands at 80 percent. This should not surprise you—medicine rarely searches for the underlying, correctable cause. But because DGL is healing in multiple ways, it has only one-third the recurrence rate of standard prescribed drugs (Morgan). With the knowledge that you are gaining here, you should be able to reduce that number to zero.

My favorite source is Rhizinate (380 mg of 4:1 deglycyrrhizinated licorice root extract and 50 mg glycine). It comes with or without fructose as a sweetener (PhytoPharmica). Two tablets should be thoroughly chewed twenty minutes before meals. Use for two to four months.

Because DGL also promotes the release of salivary compounds that stimulate growth and regeneration of stomach and intestinal cells (Bardhan 1978, Multicentre Trial 1973), it is most effective when mixed with saliva.

In the meantime, if you need an emergency antacid without aluminum in it, the same excellent-quality company makes Rhizinate combined with calcium carbonate for instant temporary relief under the name of Gastro-Relief. Chew one to four tablets as needed, but no more than thirty-two in a day. This should be a standard in your cabinet of emergency medicines.

More treatments to come in Chapter 6.

Testing for *H. pylori*

Gastroenterologists like to stick their scopes into the stomach and take a biopsy (cut out a thin piece) from the stomach wall. Long before I would allow that, I'd have the blood test. Be sure your doctor orders a quantitative antibody test though, not just a simple *H. pylori* test. The difference is important. A simple blood test will tell you whether you have antibodies to *H. Pylori* present or not, but it won't tell you if they are from an infection that you got rid of ten years ago or one that you just got two weeks ago. When you do a quantitative *H. pylori* antibody assay, however, you get a numerical amount of antibody.

If, for example, the number three weeks later is higher than the first level, it tells you that the infection is active and the bug is winning. When the level starts making a dramatic swing downward, you are conquering it. When the level of antibodies remains very low and does not fluctuate, it merely shows old infection. Just as you presumably make antibodies for life to one infection of measles, for example, the same can be true for *H. pylori*. Any time the antibody level begins to rise, especially in big jumps, then the infection is making a comeback.

Candida and *H. pylori* Are Just the Tip of the Iceberg

We've looked at the damage that Candida and *H. pylori* can do not only in the gut, but also in your whole system, ushering in symptoms galore. Well, multiply by a few hundred and you'll get an idea of how many other organisms there are that can cause any bowel problem, or trigger leaky gut, which, as you will learn, can then cause an even greater number of symptom.

Where do all these bugs come from? Newspapers and TV frequently report recalls and contaminations of products with *E. coli,* salmonella, and the like. This doesn't even begin to touch the surface of all the other bacteria, viruses, fungi, protozoa, and other parasites in our environment. With produce from all over the world in your refrigerator, you don't need to travel to contact foreign organisms.

For example, the United States Department of Agriculture (USDA) wants to define fecal matter as an acceptable part of the American diet, even though it acknowledges the dangers of food poisoning and other illnesses. "USDA pleads that condemning poultry carcasses contaminated with fecal matter during processing would work an economic hardship on the poultry industry" (Leonard). In other words, because meat and fowl handlers lobbied in government halls to save themselves money, it is acceptable to offer us progressively more contaminated proteins.

Dangerous? You bet, and even more so when you consider that everything in the gut can also get into the brain. Is food irradiation the answer? I, for one, don't think so. First of all, food irradiation destroys some vitamins and creates brand new proteins and other unique radiolytic products (URPs). These URPs have never been seen before and have not been tested.

Even worse, food irradiation does not kill all bugs. Some species of mold, like pullularia (also called *Aureobasidium*) and some species of bacteria (like the deadly *Salmonella*), are resistant to food irradiation. As a result, we have an increased chance of introducing them in greater quantities into our diets. Time is also a factor. Once a food is too old or moldy, the molds have dumped their toxins, called mycotoxins, into the food.

Irradiation can kill many types of mold but it cannot destroy the mycotoxins, which happen to be some of the most potent carcinogens known to man. When foods are slated for irradiation, it may also encourage sloppier handling, with the thought that, "Oh, well, no problem. It is going to be irradiated anyway." And more transportation and storage time (that further depletes nutrients) is needed as foods are shipped to radiation facilities, wait for processing, and are then shipped out.

Intestinal Dysbiosis: The Other Bad Bugs

Don't be put off by the term. Dsybiosis breaks down this way: dys = abnormal, as in dysfunctional, and biosis = life. The result? Abnormal life residing in the gut. This new term is meant to cover all the hundreds of other possible bacteria, viruses, fungi, protozoa, worms, and other parasites that can live in the gut and cause symptoms.

If you have a specific diagnosis of a bug, then that means you had a test ordered by your doctor to diagnose it, in which case he or she most likely has sensitivity tests and has prescribed the specific remedy for you.

Unfortunately, many folks do not have the luxury of having a test. The reasons vary: (1) they can't convince their physician to join the twenty-first century of cause-oriented medicine, (2) their physician doesn't have time to read about new tests and the evidence for them, (3) the patient can't afford a test because insurance doesn't pay for finding the cause, only blindly drugging symptoms, or (4) the HMO only condones ordering tests that every other physician does ("usual and customary"), restricting the patient to the lowest level of competency. In any of these cases, you may opt for a multipurpose bug killer for the gut.

Nonprescription Gut Bug Killers

There are some well thought out combination products that contain herbs that are safe and inhibit the growth of many of the most commonly encountered organisms, saving much time, prescription drug side effects, and money. Fortunately, by using herbal preparations that kill abnormal levels of bacteria, yeast, and protozoa, you avoid harmful antibiotics that can leave you with a yeast infection or overload an already toxic liver with newly designed chemicals.

I'll take you through just some of the ingredients of one such product, Paragard (Tyler Encapsulations, available through N.E.E.D.S.), so you can appreciate the rationale behind using it in your program to get rid of unwanted organisms or intestinal dysbiosis.

Artemisia, grapefruit seed extract, berberine, gentiana, goldenseal, quassia, garlic, and black walnut extract are examples of the many ingredients specifically chosen for their ability to eradicte the most common infectious agents in the gut. Paragard contains all of them, and one to two capsules should be taken three times a day, between meals and preferably not when you take glutamine.

One of these ingredients, extract of black walnut *(Juglans nigra),* has been used for years in folk medicine as a treatment for fungus (Tetsuro). Studies show that it is as effective as prescription antifungals (Clark). In other studies, constituent substances, like the naphthoquinones, completely inhibited fungal growth (Tripathi). Black walnut extract also has antibacterial (Krajci), antiviral, and antitumor actions (Bhargana). Other researchers have demonstrated its antibacterial action against some of the most commonly isolated causes of irritable bowel syndrome that we see: *Klebsiella, Pseudomonas, Proteus, Salmonella, Staphylococcus, Bacillus,* and *E. coli* (Tetsuro). And it is even effective against Trichophyton, which causes athlete's foot; saccharomyces, the bread yeast that we often find growing in a bloated gut; and *Cryptococcus,* as well as many species of Candida. This includes *C. tropicalis,* which is resistant to Nystatin and often grows after one has been on Nystatin unsuccessfully. (See Chapter 5.)

Another ingredient, *Allium sativa,* is better known to you as plain garlic. It, too, not only has antifungal, but also antibacterial, antitumor, and cholesterol-lowering and anticlotting properties (Hughes, Prasad, Adetumbi,

Moore). As usual, when you deal with natural remedies, the side effects tend to be beneficial. So it should come as no surprise that garlic works against amoebas, larvae, and viruses (Weber, Amonkar, Mirelman).

Berberine is an isoquinoline alkaloid found in goldenseal *(Hydrastis canadensis)* and barberry bark *(Berberis vulgaris).* For decades, it has been known to be effective in the treatment of malaria, *Entamoeba histolytica, Giardia lamblia, Trichomonas, E. coli,* colera, *Klebsiella, Salmonella,* non-specific diarrheas, and a host of other organism-caused infections, and with no toxicity (Amin, Hahn, Kaneda, Desai, Rabbani, Choudhry, Gupte, Sack, Kamat, Bhakat).

Grapefruit seed extract likewise has anti-Candidals, Geotrichum and *E. E. coli* effects (Ionescu). For its part, artemisia has been effective in dif-ficult-to-eradicate diseases like malaria, which have become resistant to high-tech medications (Trigg, Xuan-De). Again, these "antibiotics" all come without side effects because they come from the most knowledgeable biochemicst there is, Nature.

Quassia, another herbal ingredient, has also been successfully used in treating drug-resistant malaria (Kirby). It also has anti-inflammatory, anti-tumor, antiviral, and antiamoeba properties.

I could continue in this fashion and dissect all of the ingredients to show why and how they are effective against a vast majority of intestinal pathogens that cause gut symptoms, but I believe I have accomplished my purpose here. Our world is contaminated for many reasons. And the bugs that breed in contaminated substances have ready access to our intestines through the food we eat, the water we drink, and the air we breathe. Once these bugs set up housekeeping in the gut, they release abnormal amounts of gases, metabolites, and toxins that can produce any gut symptom.

If the gut is determined to get rid of them, vomiting or diarrhea result. If the toxins paralyze the gut, constipation and hemorrhoids occur. And when the bugs release their gases and metabolites you get everything from gas, pain, indigestion, and nausea to systemic symptoms of fatigue, headache, mood swings, and more. Fortunately, Nature provides remedies to harness these gut invaders. With all the clinical and scientific data available, both old and new (and I haven't even touched the surface), don't you find it in-teresting that medicine ignores Nature's remedies? Instead medicine gives top priority to drugs that do not even solve the problem in a system that re-ally is not concerned with the cause.

Remember: Always use your probiotics for a month after undergoing herbal or antibiotic treatments, since some of the good bugs can be wiped out during treatment. And once you restore the good bugs, it makes it all the more difficult for the bad bugs to get a foothold again.

The Good Bugs: Probiotics

Not all bugs are bad. Remember, not everyone gets the flu, and not everyone who kisses you when you have a cold catches it. It is not so much the virulence of the bug as it is the faulty resistance of the host. There is another factor besides the strength of your immune system that determines whether or not a bug sets up housekeeping in your gut: competition.

Nature is wonderfully orchestrated with more ingenious interwoven mechanisms than we have yet to fathom. The balance of intestinal organisms that we cannot live without is but one example. I don't need to tell you how nasty some of the more than 500 bugs in your stool are. Just smell it. But they serve to break down your food into smaller, more absorbable particles. There is a beautiful balance here, because such bugs do not cause us to rot until we die. Bacteria and fungi are what turn ashes to ashes, dust to dust.

Pro = for or promoting; biotic = life. And that's what probiotics do, promote healthy life in the gut and the whole body. They serve as competition for the bad bugs and keep them under control. Probiotics, or good bugs, also improve the integrity of the gut's immune system, fight cancer, strengthen the detoxification system, make the gut acidic through the production of lactic acid to promote digestion, produce lactase to promote the digestion of dairy products, lower cholesterol, control the overgrowth of bad bugs like Candida and invading bacteria, and even make B vitamins.

What Are the Good Bugs?

Lactobacillus acidophilus is the leader, a normal inhabitant of the large and small intestine, mouth, and vagina. *Bifidobacterium bifidum,* another good bug, accounts for 99 percent of the microflora of the large intestine of breast-fed infants, and declines in humans with age. More beneficial bugs are continually discovered, and some are what we call transient residents of the gut, but they still have multiple health benefits, like *Lactobacillus bulgaricus* and *Streptococcus thermophilus,* the two bacteria in yogurt.

So what difference do these bugs make for you? In some folks, probiotics can heal the gut, for others they can enhance their resistance to the diarrhea that travelers many times suffer, or they can improve the digestion of foods so much as to reduce food allergies. Remember as well that good bugs compete with and kill bad bugs. It's as simple as that. But every time you take antibiotics, eat a lot of junk food, have vaccinations, go through a period of severe stress, or even use herbs to kill intestinal bugs, you can distort the balance of flora in the gut. Fortunately, like so much else, you have direct control over it.

Tourista, the relentless diarrhea that ruins a vacation to foreign lands, can be prevented by taking regular daily doses of probiotics for a few weeks before leaving and all during your stay. If you think you have a healthy gut before leaving, why not play it safe and throw a bottle in your suitcase anyway. Taking probiotics once an infection starts can provide sufficient competition for the bad bugs to cause them to die off—you may avoid antibiotics entirely.

How to Select the Best Probiotics for You

A glance at any health food store shelf will reveal a confusing array of probiotics. For starters, you may be looking in the wrong place. Because they are living organisms (bacterium) that you want to reproduce and grow, setting up a lifetime of healthy housekeeping in your small intestine, they have to be alive in the bottle. Refrigeration is used to delay deterioration of things deprived of their life source. Veggies that have been cut from the ground are refrigerated, likewise, refrigeration can extend the viability or chances of a probiotic still being alive by the time you buy it.

Tablets should be avoided, as the heat generated by pressing a tablet has a greater chance of killing the bugs. Capsules are handy and provide protection for the probiotics from the harsh acid of the stomach. It is a long way to the small intestine. For others, a powdered form is better since they may not have sufficient enzymes to dissolve the capsule to release the probiotics into the small intestine. The powder form is also better for folks who cannot swallow pills. It would be best to take these between or just before meals, when the stomach acidity is less stimulated.

Is your probiotic still alive? Is it any good? To find out, take a triple or quadruple dose of what you would normally take for the product. If you get gas and bloating within a day, the organisms are growing. Don't worry—the discomfort will pass. This is the best and cheapest way to see if the bugs you have selected are still alive and in a form that allows them to flourish in your gut.

Let's look at some of my favorite brands. The following list is not exclusive, but does feature examples that I often recommend.

Vital-Dophilus (Klaire Laboratories) contains over ten billion live *Lactobacillus acidophilus* (DDS-1) per quarter teaspoon. Use one quarter to one teaspoon, one to four times a day, to just below the point of gas. You do not want to provoke symptoms, but you do want to build up the competing good flora quickly. For example, if you get extra gas with just half a teaspoon a day, cut it back to one-quarter teaspoon a day. With time you may be able to tolerate more. It takes several months to develop substantial flora. The amount of beneficial flora can be measured at any time with a special stool study, the CDSA. (See Chapter 6.) You can mix it in water, and take before or between meals.

For folks who have too much stomach acid, which kills the organisms, capsule form—with 2.5 billion organisms per capsule—is preferred. The dose again would depend on gas: one to four capsules taken one to four times a day. This form can be taken with meals, since the acid will start to dissolve the capsule.

Vital-Plex (Klaire Labs), also in powder or capsules, goes a step further, providing over 3.3 billion live organisms each of: *Lactobacillus acidophilus, Bifido bacterium bifidum* (important in colonizing the large intestine as well), and *Streptococcus faecium* (useful in diarrheal diseases) per one-quarter teaspoon.

Vital-Immune Biotic (Klaire) contains *L. acidophilus, Lactobacillus casei, Bifido longum,* as well as *Lactobacillus rhamnosus.* This one is particularly resistant to destruction from bile, has eliminated lactose intolerance for some as well as some food allergies, is strongly adherent to the gut wall, and quickly invades the large intestine as well. All three of this lab's products are as hypoallergenic as I have seen in terms of not containing other ingredients that folks with food allergies might react to.

Lactobacillus sporogenes (Thorne) has advantages over *L. acidophilus.* This is handy for those who try many different sources and routes of administration but still cannot establish a healthy level of *Lactobacillus. L. sporogenes* is acid resistant and also survives shipping better, without needing refrigeration to enhance its viability. Use one capsule three times a day.

Enterogenic Concentrate (Tyler) contains *L. acidophilus, B. bacterium bifidum, Bifido infantis,* and *Enterococcus faecium.* In addition it contains FOS that fuel the colonization of the gut with probiotics. This form of FOS is of short chain length and not as prone to intolerance as longer-chain FOS. Take one teaspoon (or two to four capsules) in a large glass of water twice daily, between meals.

Pro-Flora Concentrate (Tyler) contains eight types of probiotics. Take as above.

Kyo-Dophilus (Wakunaga) contains *L. acidophilus, B. bacterium bifidum. B. longum,* 1.5 billion cells at time of shipment; take one to four capsules two times a day. Use intestinal gas as your guide to top tolerated dose.

In a Nutshell

There are a host of nasty bugs in the world that can easily make their ways into our gut. Not only can they produce every intestinal symptom, but some of them can go on to cause cancer. Fortunately Nature, as always, has provided a balance and a cure: Good bugs fight off bad bugs and can keep them away.

CHAPTER 5

Leaky Gut Syndrome

Healing from the Inside Out

It should be no surprise: If the colon or the gut is not healthy, then the rest of the body won't be, because this is where all food and nutrients are absorbed. So even though you may have cured your gut symptoms with the techniques described in previous chapters, if you still have other symptoms and are not totally healthy, or if your gut is not yet completely well, you may have leaky gut syndrome (LGS).

How is a leaky gut born? From your months or years of food allergies, *Candida,* or anything that can inflame the gut lining. (See Table 9.) If left untreated, however, leaky gut can then precipitate anything from autoimmune diseases like multiple sclerosis, thyroiditis, lupus, and rheumatoid arthritis to fibromyalgia, chronic fatigue, brain fog, and much more.

How Food Allergies Are Born

Some folks think—mistakenly—that we are born with food allergies, and that no new allergies are possible. Because of a leaky gut, you can develop an allergy to any food at any time. Once the gut lining becomes inflamed or damaged, the spaces between gut-lining cells open up, allowing large food particles to slip through, or leak into, the bloodstream. Normally, the immune-system cells policing the blood for harmful invaders "sees" only small, tiny food particles or antigens. When they spot these new, large food particles or antigens that are foreign to the body's defense system, they attack them. Suddenly the body is producing antibodies against once harmless foods just a viciously as if they were a streptococcus bacterium. The result is allergies, developed overnight, to foods that never bothered you before. No wonder you don't stop to think that wheat, for example, could be the cause of your cramps and diarrhea when you have eaten it throughout your life in perfect freedom and without any kind of reaction.

Unfortunately, the damage that a leaky gut can cause does not stop with the production of new food allergies. Once the body starts producing attack antibodies against foods, these antibodies cruise through the bloodstream looking for prey. While doing so, the antibodies—a miniature police force of their own—can mistakenly recognize antigen-antibody receptors (like docking sites) on common body parts as similar to what they should attack. If, for example, an antibody directed toward potato recognizes a receptor on your knee cartilage that resembles it, the potato-antibody complex can attach to the knee joint. This then turns on an inflammatory reaction, suddenly causing arthritis induced by ingesting a food that used to be harmless. Every time you eat potato, you will have knee arthritis within forty-eight hours.

Or, if antibodies end up in the lungs, you develop asthma with an unsuspected food allergy as the trigger. Food allergies can precipitate symptoms in any organ at any time once the gut develops these large, leaky spaces noted above. And who would think that foods you had been accustomed to eating were now causing various symptoms throughout the body, if you did not know about the LGS and how it produces food allergies and other symptoms nearly overnight?

Some of the most incurable diseases are caused by just this mechanism, which causes the body to attack its own tissues through self-directed antibodies called autoantibodies. Most autoimmune conditions are believed to have no known cause and no effective and safe treatment. But did the doctors who came to this conclusion ever look for LGS as an initiating event? I doubt it. Rheumatoid arthritis, multiple sclerosis, thyroiditis, lupus, and coronary artery disease are just a few of the diseases that can originate with leaky gut. Happily, such conditions can be reversed in many cases.

In addition, the large, leaky spaces between gut cells allow toxins a direct route into the bloodstream. In turn, these toxins may overload the liver's work of detoxification so that everyday chemicals remain toxic. When undetoxified chemicals back up into the brain, for example, the victim can feel dizzy and unable to think straight. A person with chemical sensitivities may encounter symptoms like brain fog or mood swings when exposed to perfumes, or a new carpet or paint, perfumes or cleansers, and so on.

On the surface, it may sound like a good thing that the gut can leak. Perhaps it would enable the body to absorb more nutrients like amino acids, essential fatty acids, minerals, and vitamins. In fact, the opposite is true. In order for the body to absorb a mineral, a carrier protein must be attached to it. By hooking onto the mineral, the protein carries it through across the gut wall and into the bloodstream. But when the bowel lining is damaged by inflammation, these nutrient carrier proteins are damaged as well. The result is malabsorption; you can take in nutrients through the mouth, but they don't get absorbed. So in addition to new food and chemical allergies and autoimmune diseases, the leaky gut victim may develop mineral and vitamin deficiencies, despite taking adequate levels of them. Such nutrient deficiencies can then proceed to cause any disease we might face in a lifetime.

Bugs, Drugs, Food, and Mood Precipitate Symptoms

What common factors in your every day life can cause the inflammation that leads to LGS? Examples include

1. abnormal gut flora (e.g., uninvited bacteria, parasites, protozoa, and yeasts)
2. chemicals that irritate the gut (e.g., ingested alcohol and food additives; inhaled formaldehyde from a new carpet; or, worst of all, drugs like the NSAIDs, Motrin, Aleve, and Advil)
3. food allergens
4. stress emotions
5. genetic and acquired enzyme deficiencies (e.g., lactase deficiency, causing you to get diarrhea from dairy products, and celiac disease, which causes serious malabsorption from wheat), and more.

You might say the causes are bugs, drugs, food, and mood!

For example, when you take an antibiotic, you are at risk of developing overgrowth of antibiotic-resistant yeast or fungi (like Candida, which can mimic any symptom) or bacteria (like *Clostridia difficile,* a bacteria that can cause relentless colitis with diarrhea).

A diet high in sweets, alcohol, and caffeine can also irritate the gut lining, decreasing absorption of needed nutrients. Don't forget that processed foods with their chemical additives that can cause leaky gut are already lacking in healing nutrients, so they doubly lower nutrient status. Processed foods are a double whammy: they increase your vulnerability to leaky gut, and make healing it much harder.

Or, if a person has a lactase deficiency and ingests dairy products despite symptoms, he or she can trigger leaky gut as inflammation grows from the resulting gas and bloating. For a person with acquired celiac disease, eating barley, oats, rye, or wheat can cause a chronic inflammation of the gut lining even more serious than leakiness. When the antigen-antibody complex wipes out the absorptive fingerlike villi that line the gut, potentially fatal malabsorption can result.

Let's look more closely at one of the main causes of LGS, the classification of medications called nonsteroidal, anti-inflammatory drugs (NSAIDs), including a variety of nonprescription and prescription medications used for various types of aches, pains and sprains, arthritis, fibromyalgia, and premenstrual syndrome.

There are many over-the-counter, nonprescription drugs in the NSAIDs classification and one or more is invariably in the top ten drugs currently used by consumers. These include aspirin, ibuprofen (Motrin, Advil), and naproxen sodium (Aleve, formerly prescription Naprosyn). Tolectin, Feldene, and Voltaren are some of the prescription names. NSAIDs are a major cause of LGS because they so viciously inflame the intestinal lining, causing a widening of the spaces between cells and sometimes even hemorrhaging.

The Leaky Gut Causes a Cascade of Untreatable Symptoms

Because the leaky gut is so important, and at the same time so ignored by traditional medicine, let's make sure that, for health's sake, you are an expert on it:

- When the gut is inflamed it does not secrete digestive enzymes to digest foods properly or absorb nutrients and foods properly. The result can be indigestion with gas and bloating, called irritable bowel syndrome (IBS) by the gut specialist.
- When large food particles are absorbed, food allergies and new symptoms are created (e.g., IBS, ulcers, gallbladder disease, arthritis, or fibromyalgia).
- When the gut is inflamed, carrier proteins are damaged, so malabsorption and nutrient deficiencies occur. These deficiencies slow down the ability of the gut to heal and can cause any number of other symptoms (e.g., magnesium deficiency–induced angina or gut spasms, chromium deficiency–induced high cholesterol or sugar cravings, zinc deficiency–induced prostatitis or lack of gastric acid formation).
- When the detoxification pathways that line the gut are compromised, chemical sensitivity can arise. Furthermore, the leakage of toxins

overburdens the liver so that the body is less able to handle everyday chemicals in food, water, and air. Now many foods can cause symptoms that never did before, because the gut's detoxification system is unable to cope with the hundreds of chemical additives, dyes, colorings, preservatives, and pesticides common to our foods.

• When the gut lining is inflamed, the protective coating of gut antibodies can be lost. With loss of the secretory immunoglobulin A (sIgA), the body becomes more vulnerable to infections in the intestines from bacteria, protozoa, viruses, and yeasts (e.g., Candida), and they become resistant to treatment. Ironically the more resistant the bugs become, the more high-powered antibiotics doctors prescribe, resulting in more overgrowth of the resistant fungi (like *Candida tropicalis*). As the unwanted bugs grow, so the gut gets more inflamed and leaky initiating a vicious cycle of worsening conditions—and major cause of so many "incurable" diseases.

• When the intestinal lining is inflamed, bacteria and yeast (there are hundreds of species in the intestine) can translocate. In other words, they can pass from the gut cavity into the bloodstream and set up infection anywhere else in the body, including the brain (Berg 1988, Deitch 1987). This is often the mysterious and undiagnosed cause of infections in the teeth and gums, bones, prostate, bladder, or sinuses.

• With the formation of antibodies, the food antigens that leak across the gut wall can sometimes resemble the natural antigens on tissues. Protective antibodies will then attack the antigens, as they should, and the tissues, causing further damage. It is the very reason why autoimmune diseases begin. Lupus, multiple sclerosis, rheumatoid arthritis, myocarditis, dermatomyositis, iritis, and thyroiditis are some of the members of this ever-growing category of mysteriously "incurable" autoimmune diseases.

Now you can begin to appreciate another mechanism for how the sick get sicker when drugs mask the real cause of symptoms. For if leaky gut is chalked up to "irritable bowel disease" or "spastic colon" or "nervous colon," as it usually is, the victim is on the fast road to multiple illnesses. (See Table 10.) In reality, most IBS is really LGS in disguise, and totally curable.

Table 9. Causes of Leaky Gut Syndrome

- Intestinal dysbiosis (Candida, etc.)
- Medications (NSAIDs, etc.)
- Food allergy
- Chemical sensitivity
- Celiac disease, malabsorption
- Autoimmune disease
- Digestive insufficiencies
- Poor diet
- Nutritional deficiencies
- and more

Table 10. But The Leaky Gut Causes

- Food allergy (hence the vicious cycle)
- Chemical sensitivity
- Brain fog/toxic encephalopathy
- Autoimmune disease (RA,* etc.)
- Nutritional deficiencies
- Labelitis (CFS,* FM,* etc.)
- IBS*
- Depression
- and more

*RA = rheumatoid arthritis, CFS = chronic fatigue syndrome,
 FM = fibromyalgia, IBS = irritable bowel syndrome

Common Scenario for Leaky Gut Syndrome

An otherwise healthy person might take an antibiotic for a sore throat. The antibiotic not only goes to the throat, but also through the entire system, killing off beneficial bacteria that normally inhabit the intestines. At that point, the normally antibiotic-resistant fungi (Candida is just one example) that remain have no competition. They grow uninhibited in large numbers, inflame the intestinal lining, and cause LGS.

When large food particles leak across the intestinal lining, the victim may develop new food allergies, for example, resulting in arthritis, headaches, asthma, and other symptoms. He or she may start having gas, bloating, pain, alternating diarrhea and constipation, which is often labeled IBS or spastic colon. In reality, it is a cover-up for the honest answer, which traditional medicine usually avoids, preferring instead this well-known response: "We don't have a clue as to why you have gas, bloating, and indigestion. And we never look for environmental and nutritional causes, we don't believe in causes like food allergies or Candida, nor have we ever heard of leaky gut."

Once the leaky gut carrier proteins are damaged, however, the resulting poor absorption of minerals can lead to fatigue, inability to concentrate, multiple chemical sensitivity, depression, and other symptoms. Or, as the gut lining debilitates more, the victim can develop further infection with these fungi and other organisms. As toxicity rises, overwhelming liver detoxification pathways, a person suddenly finds himself or herself reacting to chemicals that were never bothersome before. If the brain is the chief target organ, depression or brain fog may arise here as well.

So what do people do who have arthritis, asthma, brain fog, chronic fatigue, chemical sensitivities, headaches, depression, IBS, and other conditions? They usually go to various doctors, few of whom will ever test for leaky, or hyperpermeable, gut. Instead, the doctors will prescribe a pocketful of pills; not exactly what an already overloaded detoxification system needs. In fact, it is the perfect way to make the leaky gut leakier!

Let's take a quick look now at diagnosis and treatment mechanisms for LGS, and then broaden the discussion for the most important aspects of the two. If you feel a little overwhelmed, relax. You have just learned about a medical condition that 99 percent of traditional doctors either repudiate outright or have rarely or never heard of. Congratulate yourself! You have taken a giant step toward getting and keeping yourself well.

The 8-R Outline: How to Test and Treat

Testing and treatment for LGS are done in eight phases:

1. Recognize or diagnose it before you find its cause(s).

    To diagnose LGS, do the intestinal permeability test—an easily performed urine test done at home. Your doctor merely writes a prescription for it and you call the 800 number of the lab; they will send you the kit and complete instructions. (More complete details on all tests, including interpretations of test results, can be found in Chapter 7, and all phone numbers in the Resource Guide.) If the pattern suggests malabsorption, you need to become an expert in celiac disease. (You learned about that in Chapter 2. You can also refer to my book *Wellness Against All Odds.*)

    Once you can confirm that you have LGS, you then need to find the cause. Another test, a comprehensive digestive stool analysis (CDSA—see Chapter 7), will tell you if your leaky gut is caused by Candida, Klebsiella, poor digestion, or something else.
2. Remove the cause; i.e., if there is a food allergy, or an overgrowth of Candida or other bugs, get rid of it. (Refer to Chapters 2, 3, 4.)
3. Reinoculate the beneficial bacterial flora with probiotics. (See Chapter 4.) In other words, replace the good bugs that belong in the gut and strengthen the gut's immune system.

4. Replace digestive enzymes. (See Chapter 6.)
5. Recall the total load and how chemical sensitivity can keep the gut damaged, because most detoxified chemicals pass through the gut on their way out of the body, thereby adding to the irritation of the leaky gut. It is important to learn how to reduce the total load of chemicals that the body has to detoxify. (See Chapter 6.)
6. Repair function of the gut wall with healing nutrients like fructo-oligosaccharides (FOS), L-glutamine, butyric acid, and by correcting undiagnosed nutrient deficiencies.
7. Restore good gut function by adding fiber to the diet, chewing thoroughly, drinking pure spring water, having peaceful mealtimes, getting daily physical exercise, and resolving emotional stress.
8. Rectify the cause; you also need to limit or omit NSAIDs, caffeine, and alcohol at this time. Then, you must change your diet so that you are not eating foods that you are allergic to. If you keep on with bad dietary habits, your leaky gut will recur.

So you might say the "8-Rs" recipe for healing the gut is to:

Recognize	(diagnose)
Remove	(kill bugs)
Reinoculate	(add good bugs)
Replace	(enzymes, etc.)
Recall (total load)	(FOS, L-glutamine, nutrients)
Repair	(detox the gut and life style)
Restore (function)	(fiber, chewing)
Rectify or repent	(change your dietary habits, stop taking NSAIDs, etc.)

No wonder LGS is so common. Look at all the things in our lifestyles and medical practices that cause it:

• medicating every pain with NSAIDs without finding the cause,
• using antibiotics too frequently instead of finding out why the person is so vulnerable to infection,
• eating chemicalized processed foods,
• not routinely testing for nutrient deficiencies,
• bolting down food in an unrelaxed environment.

Since leaky gut leads to the development of IBS, is it any wonder that this catch-all label is the number one gut problem? Unfortunately, the cause is rarely looked for in "modern medicine" and the drugs commonly prescribed for IBS actually guarantee that the leaky gut will get worse. For example, instead of using enzymes to promote better digestion of food into smaller particles, most IBS medications turn off gut digestive enzymes and acids. Drugs go in the opposite direction of restoring active health.

Since, as we now know, few doctors can treat LGS healthfully, it's really up to you to heal yourself. So let's look at how in more detail.

The Best Test for the Leaky Gut

The intestinal permeability test will best diagnose leaky gut. This test involves drinking a solution of two sugars: lactulose and mannitol. The gut is quite impermeable to lactulose, so it cannot simply diffuse across the gut wall. Lactose requires a carrier protein, and takes energy and work to get it across. On the other hand, mannitol should easily absorb through the gut wall without any problem.

The protocol runs as follows: drink a mixture of the two sugars in between collecting before and after urine samples. By measuring the amounts and ratios of the two sugars in the urine, we can tell how well they were absorbed, whether or not the gut is leaky, or if there is malabsorption (suggestive of celiac disease, severe food allergies, parasites, severe ulcerative colitis, and many other problems).

If the lactulose whizzes through the gut and collects in a large amount in the urine, it is a sure sign that the gut is leaky or hyperpermeable. If the mannitol does not diffuse across the gut easily, then you know that there is quite a bit of damage, and possibly serious malabsorption for certain particles as well.

If both lactuolose and mannitol are poorly absorbed, there is evidence enough for a serious six-month trial of the celiac diet. (See Chapter 2.) The diet must be not only gluten-free, but all grain-free, milk-free, and disaccharide (double sugar)-free, and it could take up to two years in serious cases of celiac or Crohn's diseases.

Crohn's disease is a serious form of colitis involving much pain, mucus, and blood. Many drugs that make the gut leakier are usually prescribed. When drugs fail, the damaged part of the colon is surgically removed. You might think following a diet is a heavy price to pay, but so is having part of your colon cut out and thrown away and wearing a bag around your waist to collect your stool for the rest of your life. In addition, this surgery can lead to decreased absorption of nutrients because of loss of the bowel; thereby making you a riskier Candidate for colon cancer and other diseases. Just one more of the vicious cycles in which the sick get sicker if they rely on drugs only.

Once you know you have LGS (as diagnosed by a positive intestinal hy-perpermeability test), it is imperative to proceed to a CDSA to find out why the gut leaks. The CDSA shows what abnormal yeasts, protozoa, and bac-teria are present and tells you if you have proper levels of digestive en-zymes. For example, if the leaky gut test reveals elevated triglycerides, fats, fatty acids, and undigested food in the stool, then you know that there are also deficient pancreatic secretions. In order to test the gut to see if there are abnormal parasites, a special Purged Parasites test is also available. (See Chapter 7.)

One reason for suspecting that you have abnormal bacteria is if you have very foul-smelling gas; or a lot of gas, or bloating, or indigestion; or alter-nating diarrhea and constipation. For these symptoms, a CDSA and seven-day Candida culture are necessary. A significant number of times I have not found Candida on CDSA but did on 7-Day Candida Culture, even though both were done at the same time.

But don't forget that the gut can be a target organ for chemical sensitiv-ity. Many times testing folks in the office for chemical sensitivity, which in-cludes minute quantities of possible allergens, will provoke their familiar intestinal spasms. (More about this in the total load section in Chapter 6.)

The Curse of Constipation

When the gut is full of bad bugs releasing noxious toxins, initial symp-toms will include diarrhea. Body wisdom says, "Get rid of this stuff." But we eat so many devitalized, fiber-poor processed foods that the body quickly loses its ability to purge itself because processed foods lack the fiber that helps hold water and bulk up the stool. Bulk is important to pro-mote gut contractility, or peristalsis, the muscular contractions that propel stool out of the colon.

In addition, processed foods lack the vital minerals that promote peri-stalsis. For example, white bleached flour has only 10 percent of the origi-nal peristalsis-promoting magnesium of whole wheat. A third cause of constipation involves the toxins of certain intestinal bugs that actually par-alyze peristalsis by intoxicaing its related nerves. When peristaltic waves no longer push food along, constipation results. The longer food sits rotting in the constipated colon, the more it will release bowel-paralyzing toxins. Once again we note the vicious cycle: the sick get sicker.

Certainly one of the first things you must do here is to get the food within you moving again. As long as there are putrefactive wastes sitting on the gut wall day in and day out, the wall will weaken. Your general strength can also suffer as the build up of toxins enters the system, triggering achiness, fatigue, and mood swings. In addition, as the weak areas of the gut wall balloon out you will develop diverticulitis. As these pockets now collect bacteria and become infected, antibiotics are called in to help. The result is yeast overgrowth and leaky gut. Had enough? I sure hope so. Because constipation is a sure road to ill health.

Enter the vitamin C flush or The Pure Body Program as described below to nip your constipation in the bud!

Vitamin C Flush

Take one heaping teaspoonful of Klaire Lab's Ultra Fine Ascorbic Acid Powder in a large eight-ounce glass of water. Repeat this every hour until you get diarrhea. Once you do, cut back to a total daily dose where there is no diarrhea, just a normal daily movement or two.

Because vitamin C is highly acidic and can dissolve tooth enamel, don't forget to rinse your teeth after the flush. The vitamin C flush is one of the safest and most healthful cures for constipation. If after five days there is no response, see your physician. Of course, it goes without saying that if you are still on a bad diet, the vitamin C flush will not work as well as it should or will not work at all.

The Pure Body Program

An alternative or addition to the vitamin C flush is the Pure Body Program (Pure Body Institute), consisting of two bottles. The first bottle, called Nature's Cleansing Program: Whole Body, contains herbs to detoxify, heal, and cleanse the bowel; take three to seven tablets twice a day a half hour before meals with a large glass of water. The second bottle, called Nature's Cleansing Program: Colon, contains herbs to "hoe out" the gut, removing concretions of old stool and mucus; take one to three tablets at the same time but with another large glass of water one to four times a day.

The Magnesium Flush

Folks are often so low in magnesium from eating processed foods (the average American diet does not even provide half of your daily requirement) that the gut is in constant spasm, resulting in constipation, sometimes alternating with bouts of spastic diarrhea. An easy way to diagnose and treat the problem is to take one teaspoon of liquid 18% Magnesium Solution (Ecologic Formulas, or ARG) two to three times a day in a large glass of water for a week. You can improve its chances of working by adding manganese picolinate 20 milligrams (Thorne) once a day to your nutrients, as it makes a long-standing deficiency bounce back quicker for many people. (Stop if stools are too loose or any other adverse symptoms occur.) As a result, you will sleep better; feel less edgy or depressed; and experience less back spasms, headaches, or other symptoms of magnesium deficiency.

Healing the Leaky Gut

Here is a first-line treatment to which the majority of people respond. For those who do not respond positively, you will need to work up a more personalized program with your physician.

Again, the first step in treating the leaky gut is finding out why it leaks. Hidden food allergy is a major cause, and by following the rare food diagnostic diet (see Chapter 2) you'll be able to figure out your hidden food allergies.

Next comes an unsuspected infection of the gut, like Candida overgrowth from years of sporadic antibiotics, lots of sweets, or bacterial or protozoa infections stemming from eating out, contaminated municipal waters, and more. It is imperative to obtain a test of the stool to determine if parasites, bacteria, protozoa, or fungi (yeasts or molds) are present. Then you can use the protocols in Chapters 3 and 4 to kill these organisms.

What if your doctor balks at ordering a test to determine if you have leaky gut, *Candida,* or food allergies? You may be among the lucky ones who can use a shotgun approach. By this I mean using a preparation that has potent herbs to kill the most commonly encountered bugs. Paragard (Tyler or N.E.E.D.S.) contains time-honored herbs to eradicate the most commonly encountered abnormal organisms ("bugs") in the gut. (More on the ingredients and how to take it in Chapter 4.)

Another alternative to antibiotics is using herbs known to discourage the growth of all sorts of unwanted intestinal bugs. Citramesia (Ecologic Formulas) contains 400 milligrams of *Artemisia annua,* an herb that even kills malaria parasites; 100 milligrams of grapefruit seed extract, known for its anti-Candida and other microbial-killing powers; and echinacea, an immune-boosting herb.

Having identified the cause of your leaky gut, you can use glutamine to heal it. In fact, glutamine is so healthful to the gut that it actually inhibits radiation-induced colitis. In other words, when people have cancer of the abdomen, they often undergo radiation to the abdomen, which is at times a very dangerous procedure. Cases have been reported, for example, where, as a side effect of successful radiation therapy, the patient has died because the radiation also destroyed the gut. Glutamine, however, even in small doses of 500 milligrams three times a day, will shield the gut from radiation damage. This is potent proof of the protection that glutamine provides, and which is mainly found in the small bowel.

Start with a teaspoon of pure powdered L-glutamine (Thorne, Jarrow, ARG) 5 grams, twice a day in water, later reducing it. There must be no food in the stomach for one to two hours before and after taking it, as acid destroys its activity. If preferred, it comes as L-Glutamine 1000 milligram pharmaceutical grade tablets (Jarrow) or L-Glutamine 500 milligram tablets (Bio-Tech). If you do better with smaller doses than normal, take one to five tablets twice a day in water and between meals (no food or drink an hour before or after). Very infrequently, glutamine can trigger a depressive reaction in the brain, so start low if you are prone to such a reaction.

L-glutamine is also contained in combination with other beneficial ingredients for healing the gut, like phosphatidylcholine and gamma linolenic acid, both crucial for repair of gut cell membranes, the site of damage.

Enterogenic Factor (Tyler) is an additional combination therapeutic that contains FOS. These are the very nutrients that intestinal cells need in order to regenerate as they heal. Enterogenic Factor also contains the probiotics otherwise known as the beneficial gut flora, or good bugs. Replacing gut flora with the proper, beneficial bacteria does many things, from promoting healing of the leaky gut, to stopping the leaking (translocation or migration) of nasty bugs directly into the bloodstream to other organs. Without the good bugs to protect the wall, you increase the chances of gut bacteria setting up housekeeping in the prostate or, for that matter, in a tooth root.

When the gut is leaky, it does not secrete its digestive juices well. This leads to poorly digested food particles leaking across the gut wall into the blood. One way to stop this vicious cycle is to add digestive enzymes to your diet. Such enzymes will facilitate your capacity to break down foods into smaller particles that the immune system does not react against with destructive antibiodies. As you read in Chapter 1, there are many types of digestive enzymes available in powerful combinations. Similase (Tyler), with a dose of one to four capsules with meals, is an excellent choice, as is Biogest (Thorne), in the same dose. (For more details and options, see Chapter 6.)

Don't get overwhelmed by the number of digestive enzyme combinations available and all that you might need. As you can appreciate, if the cause of your leaky gut is simple, like the use of NSAIDs or overgrowth of Candida, stopping the use of NSAIDs or killing the Candida may improve the leaky gut enough so that you may only need L-glutamine two to three times a day between meals, for a month or two. However, if the gut is more damaged or resistant to healing, you will need to do a lot more of the 8-R program.

A logical package for a newcomer who has a leaky gut, as medically documented, is the Tyler Program:

To kill bad bugs	Paragard (two capsules two to three times a day between meals)
To put the good bugs back in	Enterogenic concentrate (one teaspoon three times a day between meals)
To heal the gut wall	Permeability factors (one to two capsules three times a day between meals)
To restore digestion	Similase (one to four with meals)

Begin slowly begin with one substance for a few days, then add on the next, reaching as many as your tests or your gut-level feeling tell you that you need in order to heal. Perhaps you would only need one product, or only one of each product. We are all different. There are others you could take, but the Tyler Program works for the vast majority of people.

Other products to possibly add to the Tyler Program include the following:

To add fiber to the gut	Fiber Formula (one to four twice a day)
To improve detoxification	Detoxification Factors (one to two twice a day)
To correct nutrient deficiencies	OxyPerm (one twice a day) MultiPlex-1 without Iron (one to two a day)

What you will take depends entirely on the severity of your condition. The beauty of it all is that the condition is curable. And don't be disillusioned if you cannot take all the substances listed. Pick out what you think might be important, use it, and evaluate the effect. Don't rely on capsules alone, however, without changing your diet.

As there are many ways in which to heal, there are many agents that promote healing. You may start with only one item and be successful or you may need several items taken together.

Another program designed to heal the gut is the HealthComm Program, which involves taking Ultra Clear, a powdered, hypoallergenic supplement that contains nutrients to sustain you as well as to heal the gut. Because of its low antigenicity (low chance of developing allergies to it) and many healing nutrients as well as some calories, it can sustain you if you choose to rest your gut by taking no food for a few days. Should symptoms suddenly vanish, it is a sure sign that food allergy is one of the culprits. Merely mix two heaping tablespoonfuls in water and drink it three to five times a day. If you you choose to eat during this time, feel free to do so but in this fashion: Make each meal out of one food at a time, so you can be sure of whether or not you are allergic to that food.

Peeling Back the Layers of Causes

I've been fortunate to see folks from all over the country who have gotten themselves markedly better just by following the steps and programs mentioned. Thirty years ago when I graduated from medical school, my classmates and I were not trained in how to teach the patient how to get well. Nor is such training a priority today. Yet I never cease to be amazed at how much healing the average person is capable of on his or her own, even after all medical regimens offered have failed. It is indeed a wonderful thing for a doctor to hear, as one patient put it: "I can't believe it. I've accomplished in a few weeks on my own what my seven doctors couldn't help me with over the last four years!"

Remember as well that if you choose a shotgun treatment and do not succeed immediately, abandon it and start over, this time the right way with a proper diagnosis and an individualized prescribed treatment. Likewise, when you have done any treatment for a month or more without results, go back to square one. Determine precisely what is wrong with your bowel and reformat your program accordingly.

For example, say you did the leaky-gut test, found out it was leaky, and decided to work on the many food allergies that you know you have. By doing a CDSA you might have found that you had a gut full of yeast, or a bacteria called Proteus that is sustaining the inflammation despite your best efforts. Or say you did a CDSA, found Klebsiella, and began treatments specifically for Klebsiella.

Sometimes finding the cause is like peeling the layers of an onion. If the CDSA reveals overgrowth of Candida and you treat it but are still sick, look again. A follow-up CDSA may show an overgrowth of klebsiella had been masked by the previous Candida overgrowth. Often, patients have had to peel back as many as three and four layers to discover all the causes of their symptoms.

At the very least, it is important to do a leaky-gut test, which can also identify a more threatening condition, like a malabsorption—which will continue to make your life miserable until you treat it. In that case, you might want to do a blood test for antigliadin and antigluten antibodies that help diagnose celiac disease, or gluten enteropathy, and to start a strict gluten-free diet.

There is much more you could do to get well, but which may require a specialist. For example, short chain fatty acids, like butyric acid, help the large intestine to heal. In fact, butyric acid is such an important nutrient that it, like vitamin A and other nutrients, has caused cancerous cells to re-differentiate, or return to normal. As a result, butyric acid is a must in conditions like ulcerative colitis, Crohn's disease, and cancer, not to mention intestinal hyperpermeability, or leaky gut. Butyric acid retention enemas (Tyler) are available and should be taken at home (directions included) one to three times daily. But much easier for beginners is to take Cal-Mag Butyrate (Ecologic Formulas), one to six capsules, after meals. I'll give you lots of other ideas in the next chapter.

As usual, just as important as what you take in, is what you don't take in. A leaky gut, for example, may be damaged by alcohol; NSAIDs; H2-blockers and other medications; chemotherapy; fasting; food allergies; gluten enteropathy, or celiac disease; inhaled pesticides; nonorganic pesticided and chemically laden food; parasites; or abnormal amounts of certain bacteria, fungi, or yeast. If you still need your morning coffee, your afternoon snack of junk food, and your evening alcoholic drink, you may retard healing indefinitely.

And do not ignore common sense. If you spend time chewing your food (ten to fifty times a mouthful), you will promote better absorption. Mixing food well with saliva takes some of the work away from the gut. And when you really taste some of the food you eat, you may opt for more "real" food.

As well as exercising your jaws, don't neglect to exercise the muscles surrounding the gut. Learn yoga stretches or play tennis, or just enjoy a daily walk with a friend.

If at any time you are stuck at a plateau and not getting better, it is best to have a blood test for minerals and fatty acids, as deficiencies can hold up healing indefinitely. For example, if you do not have enough hydrochloric acid, you cannot absorb all the needed nutrients (Recker). Unfortunately, with H2-blocker medicines such as Tagamet (cimetidine), Axid (nizatidine), Zantac (ranitidine), and Pepcid (famotidine) now available over the counter, many more innocent people are turning off their acid without considering the consequences.

Hold Those Nutrients

While attempting to heal the gut, it is a good idea to hold off on your nutrient corrections for a while. You'll get more for your money by correcting nutrient deficiencies once the gut is more efficient at absorbing and utilizing your nutrients. If nutrients are just going to pass through unused, why take them until the gut is healed, or at least partially better?

It may also turn out that, by trying to correct nutrient deficiencies while healing your gut, you will irritate it further, waste money, and drive yourself crazy with trying to do everything at once. There is only so much work that you or your gut can do in a day. So, heal your gut first and then proceed to correcting nutrient deficiencies, or take the nutrients only two days a week while you are in the early stages of healing.

There is, however, one nutrient now available that could be very beneficial to healing the gut: liquid ubiquinone, or coenzyme Q10; called OptiQ-100 (Phillips Nutritionals), it should be taken in doses as high as one to two teaspoons two to three times a day. Why is this the case with OptiQ-100 and not other nutrients?

- First, it is easily absorbed,
- second, it sops up free radicals that retard healing (Landi, Beyer), and
- third, it provides the intracellular (inside the cell) energy needed to promote protective mucus secretion and rapid cell growth for healing an ulcer, gastritis, and LGS (Salim Kohli, Gaby).

There are many other healing tools for the gut, but those just mentioned are excellent basic starters, and for the majority, all that you'll need. On the flip side, there are causes of some complexity, which require the simpler programs just to calm your system down, enabling you to identify the primary cause. (More on that in Chapter 6.)

Beyond the Leaky Gut: Total Load

Total load is another important concept that traditional medicine ignores. Yet, until total load is addressed, it is another potent reason why many folks will never get better. Examining total load means looking for all the things that contribute to symptoms.

If, for example, the cause of your irritable bowel symptoms is Candida and food allergy, but you only treat Candida, you won't get better, even though the Candida is gone. In more complicated cases there may also be leaky gut, nutrient deficiencies, parasites, or a grouchy spouse.

Another reason for failure is fixation. Beware getting fixated on the wrong diagnosis! Whenever you focus exclusively on one problem and find you are stuck and not healing, stop and consider what may be holding you back. For example, you can be very diligent about killing yeast only to find that you are not that much better, even though you have proven that you have an overgrowth. This signifies that you must heal something else before you can progress to better health. A common need is to resolve nutrient deficiencies in the detoxification pathways. (See Chapter 6.)

Listen to your body. It is your best teacher, because it usually expresses priorities as to what it wants healed first. And each person's is different. The fault may lie in the immune system, in the detoxification system, or in the gut wall, whose internal defense system is too depleted of nutrients. Extremely helpful at this juncture, is knowing your fatty acid and red blood cell mineral status. After identifying and correcting deficiencies, if there is still a problem, look at your detox status (comprehensive detox panel). Don't get blindly fixated on a yeast program for years on end, as I have seen many folks do. Look at what else is missing in your total load to enable you to be healthy enough so that your body can heal itself.

In terms of detoxification, recall that the gut is the main area where the body dumps chemicals it has detoxified from food, water, and air. Should the detox system be overworked, say from a diet high in processed foods, or from living or working in a new or recently renovated building, or from pesticiding or painting at home, its capacity to do its job may be compromised—which can then also stress out the liver—something you don't want to happen.

Still toxic bile, of course, as it returns to the gut, will irritate and inflame it, perpetuating leakiness. But if the daily detoxification work that your body and gut have to do is lessened, the gut has a better chance of healing. I hope you can now appreciate why the chemical overload in your living and working environments suddenly becomes very important to the rest of your health. This is where environmental controls, antioxidants, and detox enemas, as detailed in Chapter 6, can help you heal faster.

Many areas of "modern" living contribute to your unseen total load—you cannot always deal with all of them, nor do you have to in order to get well. But by increasing your knowledge about the many unseen dangers you may encouter you do have a better chance of defending yourself and choosing those parts of the total load that you can do something about. **Bottom line:** reduce your body's total load sufficiently to enable it to heal itself.

Let's look again at an example of an unseen technology that silently contributes to your total load: irradiated foods. Often without stating so on their labels, most shrimp, herbs, potatoes, and other products are nearly routinely irradiated. As a result, many problems are created:

- The ionizing radiation turns some of the food constituents into new entities, called unique radiolytic products (URPs). These have never been seen before and have not been tested. They are mutagens, substances capable of changing our genetics and producing cancer. Many URPs are cytotoxic, or toxic to cells.
- The irradiation of foods also lowers the vitamin content by actually destroying some of the vitamins.
- Yet irradiation does not do a thing to inactivate the toxins produced by molds in foods. These mold toxins (mycotoxins) like aflatoxin A1, are some of the most potent causes of cancer known to scientists.
- Also some species of salmonella are radiation-resistant, as are some species of mold, like pullularia (also called Aureobasidium). And if

you have a leaky gut, guess what? These radiation-resistant fungi and their toxins can pass directly from the gut into the bloodstream (called translocation) and even into the brain.

This is just one reason why you need an ongoing program to keep yourself informed about your environment. By avoiding irradiated foods (as, for example, milk or chicken displayed without refrigeration) or when you see the tiny radura logo on a product, you are taking another step forward in reducing your total load of contaminants for the gut to detoxify.

It may still seem strange to you that the air in your house has a bearing on healing your gut or any other condition, but it does. It even has an immense bearing on whether or not you get cancer or any other disease. Clean air, food, and water are paramount to healing and staying well.

In a Nutshell

Lets recap some essential facts. First, at bare minimum, one out of four people has irritable bowel syndrome (IBS). In other words, the gut is not healthy and doctors are stumped. Much of it can be due to a leaky gut.

If the IBS is not due to leaky gut, and if left untreated or merely medicated, it can eventually cause leaky gut. This, in turn can trigger an avalanche of symptoms anywhere in the body, symptoms which usually defy diagnosis, much less treatment. When leaky gut triggers symptoms that seem totally unrelated to the gut, like serious depression or autoimmune diseases, suddenly the gut is no longer the focus. The presence of more demanding symptoms also decreases any chance that you or your doctor will diagnose the underlying leaky gut.

Meanwhile, everything in the gut can make its way into the blood and the brain (Kare), causing dizziness, depression, and other symptoms. And all because we live in a society in which people take medications to alleviate gut symptoms and then forget about them; a society in which television ads advise you to take medications even before you go out and intentionally destroy your gut with unhealthy food and drink.

You either have leaky gut or you do not. Yet the mere presence of gut symptoms indicates that even if you do not yet have it, you could, and most likely will, if you do not learn the cause of your symptoms and correct them, immediately. You can have your doctor order the leaky-gut test, or you can use the therapies discussed in this chapter as you seek to improve in your condition.

CHAPTER 6

Finding the Best Treatment for You, or Fixing What's Broken

Gut-Level Medicine

"Wait a minute. Did I miss a step?" you ask. You know that a classic medical workup involves a history of the illness, then a physical, then a barrage of blood tests and/or X rays. "Can I jump into treatment before all the diagnostic tests?" That's easy—the answer is *yes*. For starters:

1. Many symptoms can be treated simply and inexpensively and with little or no side effects by using natural remedies. For example, giving up processed foods, coffee, and alcohol, and taking deglycyrrhized licorice or DGL (Rhizinate) may cure your chronic indigestion.
2. When using the cause-versus-drug approach, the diagnostic process itself can also be a treatment. For example, finding hidden food allergies with the diagnostic diet allows you to eliminate foods you are allergic to.
3. Most folks have already had a conventional workup to rule out physical lesions like ulcers, Crohn's disease, or cancer.
4. If all else fails, please go to the next chapter and get the proper diagnostic tests done.

For each category, I'll begin with the simpler remedies that help a majority of folks and progress to more sophisticated combinations for more resistant cases. But never lose sight of the fact that you are an *individual*. You can do as many or as few of the remedies as you feel you need. Judge your success by your own results. And if your health does not improve, know that you need to explore more options as presented.

For example, take one hundred folks with indigestion. Some benefit immediately just by cutting out their junk food, coffee, alcohol, or cigarettes. In the meantime, the safe and effective herbal DGL (Rhizinate) can provide safe symptomatic and therapeutic relief along the way.

Of course, I don't expect you to drop all your bad habits in one day. In fact, you may keep some of them for some time. If, for example, you are going through a particularly stressful period in your life and have cut out the soda, junk food, and alcohol, but simply can't quit smoking, then keep the cigarettes for now. Give yourself a well-deserved pat on the back for what you have accomplished and enjoy the fruits of your labor. Every positive step you take toward wellness is better than not having taken it. Even if it does not bring that final relief of symptoms you so much desire, it is one more part of your total load removed, one more step toward health, one more step toward cure.

As your symptoms start melting away with every positive step you take, you will feel progressively more energetic. Feeling well for the first time in your life may also empower you to break some controlling addictions. So don't rush it if your life is not yet ready for a particular stage.

If at any time you feel worse, or are not getting any better, it is certainly time to return to your doctor for the appropriate tests. To simplify the short-term need for symptomatic relief while you uncover the cause of your symptoms, see Table 13 for a list of natural remedies that you can stock your nonmedicine chest with for a quick fix.

In Chapter 7, I have provided explanations for all tests: why and when you should have them and what they measure. You may very well need this information, especially if you must ask your doctor to order certain tests and if he or she is unfamiliar with nondrug, nontoxic treatments for the ailments you suffer from.

Fortunately, there is new awareness among a small, but growing number of physicians who seek to cure causes, not only symptoms. You can recognize such physicians by how well they explain their methods to you and by the printed handouts and booklets they give you or that they suggest you read. They know that the smarter you are, the better health you will have.

Treatments for GI Conditions

Caveats: When should you stop any symptomatic treatment?—within a few days of the disappearance of symptoms. If symptoms recur, then return to your treatment while you intensify your quest for the cause. Remember, your goal is not to need ongoing treatment, but to become free of symptoms and treatments. Another time to stop any treatment is if you feel *worse*. Feeling worse could be a sign that you are allergic to an ingredient or have not gone as far as you need to to isolate the real underlying cause.

But combination diagnostic and therapeutic regimens, like the yeast program, do require patience for the healing to occur. Although you may feel much better than you did within a few days or weeks of starting your regimen, don't stop there—continue it for one to three months. **Remember:** your multiple purpose here includes reducing the amount of an unwanted fungus, encouraging the growth of the good bugs once again, and allowing the gut to heal after such a long time of inflammation driven by undiagnosed infection.

Although I will discuss the most common symptoms for each diagnosis, know also that folks have a spectrum of symptoms. One person with irritable bowel syndrome (IBS) may have only a feeling of gas and bloating after every meal, mimicking a Candida overgrowth. Another may have intense pain with cramps and diarrhea so severe they can mimic Crohn's disease, one of the more severe types of colitis.

In addition, some folks are what we call the "outlyers." Although their symptoms are not unlike those common to a specific disease, theirs are more unusual and make physicians suspect something entirely different. Other folks are constantly evolving, with symptoms changing from week to week, making diagnosis all the more difficult.

In terms of contraindications for any protocols, basic tenets apply across the board: If you become worse or are sensitive to any of the ingredients, discontinue the path you are on and fine-tune your diagnosis before you proceed. We are all biochemically unique.

In terms of products, I have only selected those from top companies that I have known and used, many for over two decades. In fact, I can't give the products I do recommend any higher endorsement than saying that they work well and safely. Although several manufacturers, knowing of my use of their products, have asked me to take on the role of paid consultant or paid spokesperson for them, or to sell the products directly to my patients, I have scrupulously avoided any behavior which would compromise my integrity as a medical practitioner and healer.

In terms of side effects for any of the protocols offered her, they tend to be far fewer than for drugs. Why? For the most part, they are natural remedies that promote healing rather than turning off normal body functions. Often the worst "side effect" is really the die-off. You recall from the Candida section that the release of toxins from killed fungi can duplicate all of your worst symptoms for several days. But you can greatly reduce or entirely eliminate this by reducing the numbers of fungi before treatment with the milk of magnesia purge as described.

You are already aware of some of the treatments I will recommend:

- diagnosing hidden food allergies with the diagnostic diet (see Chapter 2),
- treating Candida or using the Paragard protocol (see Chapter 3),
- treating *H. pylori,* using a probiotic protocol, intestinal dysbiosis protocol, or the DGL, or Rhizinate, protocol (see Chapter 4),
- for treating the leaky gut, the vitamin C flush, or the Pure Body protocol (see Chapter 5)

Refer back to the corresponding sections to refresh your memory when you need to. (See Table 12 for a summary of treatments.) These protocols form the core of the solutions that enable many folks to heal their gut disease. Details of other protocols with an asterisk (*) will be found later in this chapter.

All tests are described in Chapter 7. For product sources, the toll-free numbers of companies are in the Resource Guide. N.E.E.D.S. also carries everything listed in this book, which is especially useful since some suppliers sell only in huge quantities or to professionals or to retailers. So let's get you well!

Mouth Sores, Canker Sores, Mouth Ulcers

Hidden food allergies, not viruses, are the most common cause of mouth sores, and the same goes to canker sores and mouth ulcers. For example, a very common cause of mouth sores is a recent increase in the amount of acidic foods that you eat, such as citrus, vinegars, tomatoes, strawberries,

Table 11. Quick Guide to Finding the Protocols in Previous Chapters

Protocol	Chapter
Diagnostic diet for hidden food allergies	2
Candida	3
Paragard	3
H. pylori	4
Probiotic	4
Intestinal dysbiosis (unwanted gut bugs)	4
DGL (Rhizinate)	4
Leaky gut syndrome	5
Pure Body Program	5
Vitamin C flush	5
Magnesium flush	5

and similar foods, especially if they are seasonal. Being able to turn on and off mouth sores within forty-eight hours of consuming the suspected food is a great clue to what's causing your mouth sore.

If however, your sores are due to a virus, and you prefer to guess that that's the case, then you have a good chance of nipping them in the bud. As soon as you feel a sore coming on, use a packet of Biopro-A Thymic, under the tongue for as long as you can hold it, every three to six hours. Often this will stop the virus from persisting days and weeks longer as they sometimes do. To increase your chances of success, do the detox enema* daily and the vitamin C flush or the detox cocktail* three to five times a day. All of these serve to boost the immune system's ability to fight a virus, should that be the cause. Remember the DGL (Rhizinate) protocol also has antiviral properties and clears cold sores as well.

Another option is to cleanse the bowel with chlorophyll and use one of nature's antibiotics, garlic. Kyo-Green (Wakunaga), one to two heaping tablespoons in a large glass of water, three to six times a day, plus Kyolic (Wakunaga), two to three capsules, two to three times a day would accomplish this.

You could do any or all of these, but if cold sores keep recurring, you need to find the food allergy source and/or what nutrients you are deficient in that make you so vulnerable to attack. Again, all nutrient tests are in Chapter 7.

If you already have a low acid and very healthful diet and suspect the cause is viral, try Tea Tree Oil (Gold Mine Natural Food or N.E.E.D.S. catalogs) dropped on the lesion thrice daily with a Q-tip; dilute it with water if it is too strong for you. You will feel a burning sensation but that will pass.

An alternative multipurpose antiviral/antibiotic is Water Oz Mineral Water Silver (Water Oz), one teaspoonful, taken daily, should be held in the mouth on the lesion (tilt head appropriately) a few minutes, then swallowed.

Halitosis

Bad breath, or nasty odors from the mouth, has many causes from undetected infection in the sinuses, teeth, or gums, to insufficient use of a water pick and dental floss. A gut full of bad bugs or the rotting of poorly chewed, poorly digested foods are also prime causes.

Be sure you do not have Candida, need digestive enzymes*, or need probiotics. A simple solution that addresses all three would be to take Paragard or Kyolic to kill bugs, Similase or Biogest to boost enzymes, and VitalPlex or Kyo-dophilus to restore the good bugs. There are scores of other options. I'm merely trying to give you a feel for how you might formulate your plan.

Food allergy and/or eating too much dead food is a common cause of halitosis, as is insufficient chewing. The diagnostic or the Candida diet, often solves the problem. A badly coated tongue is a sure sign of toxicity, and can come from a polluted bowel or Candida.

Should a polluted bowel (intestinal dysbiosis) be your problem, then a simple Pure Body Program* or fasting will be helpful.

Nausea and Vomiting

Pregnant women commonly feel nauseous and prone to vomit. Known medically as hyperemesis gravidarum, nausea of pregnancy, a simple lack of vitamin B_6 is often the cause. To supplement, I recommend vitamin B_6 in liquid form from Carlson Laboratories, 200 milligrams per teaspoon, so the dose can be easily titrated to need (starting with a lower dose and working up slowly every few days until you stop the symptom or reach top dose); usually 100 milligrams one to three times a day will solve the problem. It would be best to have your B_6 blood level and that of other nutrients as well, measured by your gynecologist, since two lives depend on this. Whatever you take, always check with your gynecologist/obstetrician, the rightful captain of the ship, first. Treating pregnant people is beyond the scope of this book. If you are not pregnant, B_6 deficiency is not a likely cause of nausea.

Aside from pregnancy, there are other causes and cures for that queasy feeling in the pit of the stomach. If the nausea or vomiting is due to sea or motion sickness, ginger root works well, either as an infusion (tea) or in tablet, liquid, or capsule form as GingerMax (PhytoPharmica).

If your nausea and vomiting may be due to a brain tumor or inner-ear infection, get it diagnosed. In other words, if you explore suggestions here without success, just remember that the cause of your symptoms may be something other than what you believe it is—and that requires proper diagnosis and treatment.

Allergy, of course, is a very common cause of nausea, with foods, dusts, molds, pollens, and environmental chemicals as triggers. To identify the culprits you will need to do the diagnostic diet and establish some measure of control over common environmental contaminants*.

If nausea is a reaction to something you ate recently, get rid of it as soon as possible. One teaspoon of Epsom salts or ipecac (from a pharmacy) in a large glass of water will induce vomiting, as will a finger down the throat. When the body tells you to get rid of something you just ate, don't argue. Just do it. To ignore Mother Nature for the sake of convenience or to avoid social embarassment may mean paying in spades later on. A hepatitis-laden raw oyster or a bad clam at a party could change your life.

Nearly all medications, even supplements, have the potential to cause nausea. Check with your doctor before stopping prescribed medications for a few days' trial to determine if they are the cause of your nausea.

Hiatus Hernia, Gastroesophageal Reflux Disease (GERD), Acid Heartburn, Reflux Esophagitis

The symptoms of the above conditions, all of which are similar, can range from nausea, chest pain, chest burning to a feeling of fullness or of undigested food. Because they can mimic a heart attack, always be cautious and rule that out first. Sometimes coughing or asthma at night will be the only symptoms of reflux.

The diaphragm is a thick, flat muscle that separates the lungs from the gut. There is a tiny hole in the diaphragm that the esophagus (the main tube from the mouth to the stomach) slips through. Sometimes, being overweight or heavy lifting can cause the muscles around this hole to be torn. If enough damage has occurred, the opening becomes sloppy and a corner of the stomach slides up into the lung area. If it gets trapped there, it can cause such severe pain that you would swear you were having a heart attack.

Another problem arises when the stomach partly slides up into the lung side of the diaphragm. In order to accomplish this, the valve between the esophagus and stomach has to tear loose from its connection. With the loss of the muscular attachment and control, the valve becomes loose, or sloppy. Now the strong acid from the stomach, and even some of the undigested food, can slide up into the esophagus. Since the delicate lining of the esophagus was never meant to tolerate acid, it burns. With the esophagus passing right in front of the heart, no wonder this is called heartburn.

If the valve is truly leaky and is the cause of the backwash, or reflux, of stomach acid into the esophagus, put a cement block under each of the legs at the of the bed so that it is on a slant. This discourages backwash up into the esophagus as you sleep.

Do not eat large meals that stretch out the valve, but small frequent meals, and do not eat for three hours before going to bed. See the Parasympathetic protocol* for more detailed help here.

Make sure you have ruled out food allergy and Candida, since these are often the real culprits, despite X ray findings to the contrary. As I stated previously, we know this to be true by virtue of this fact: Once folks have treated their Candida or food allergy, their symptoms usually disappear. This is so despite an X ray that reveals a hiatus hernia, albeit totally aymptomatic, and that does not require you to elevate the head of your bed for relief.

If you have a large and resistant herniation and are contemplating surgery, on the other hand, you may want to do a trial of natural-source antacid, made from aloe vera. Use Pure Aloe Vera (Klaire), one to two tablespoons or Aloe Gel Caps (Carlson) before bedtime and as needed through the night. For it is the leaking of gastric juice into the delicate esophagus that creates the burning.

Do not use spearmint or peppermint, as these carminatives (digestive stimulants) actually lower the pressure in the valve and can make the reflux worse. On the flip side, licorice root preparations containing DGL help normalize the pressure and stimulate protective mucus. Again, use the Rhizinate protocol.

Or use any of the remedies below for gastritis, especially Gastro-Relief (PhytoPharmica), because it contains calcium carbonate as a safe, aluminum-free antacid, as well as the healing DGL of Rhizinate.

Gastritis, Heartburn, Esophagitis, Nonulcer Dyspepsia (NUD), Dyspepsia, Acid Indigestion

Gastritis, heartburn, esophagitis, nonulcer dyspepsia (NUD), and acid indigestion are similar in their effects: With minor variations they make your gut feel lousy.

Know as well that symptoms can overlap with hiatus hernia in some folks or with gallbladder disease in other folks. These include a dull aching, uncomfortable fullness, or the feeling that everything you've eaten is sitting there and ballooning. Or they can manifest as overt burning or pain, or both, with or without nausea and vomiting.

Food allergy or overload (glutinous overeating and eating processed foods) are the most common causes. It goes without saying that you should avoid processed foods, known allergens, and difficult-to-digest foods and food combinations. Peaceful eating circumstances, thorough chewing, and not diluting what digestive acids you do have with too much liquid are also important helpmates here. Save drinking for after dinner and rely on copious chewing to take its place. The only time you want to drink several glasses of water with meals is to help you decide if you actually feel better due to the fact that water dilutes excess acid.

Therapeutic protocols for gastritis and company include:

- *H. pylori* protocol. This bug can be the sole cause of these symptoms.
- Candida protocol. Likewise, Candida can be the sole cause of symptoms.
- Digestive enzymes protocol. Some folks just need a boost of their digestive enzymes.

- Sometimes relief can be a simple as drinking ginger tea, best made by grating a teaspoon of fresh ginger into a tea ball, then steeping it in a teapot of hot water for ten minutes. Sip this throughout the day. Chamomile is another soothing tea.
- An antacid from organic aloe vera juice, Pure Aloe Vera (Klaire) as above.
- Carlson's Aloe Gel caps, which are equivalent to a cup of juice.
- DGL (Rhizinate) protocol, thoroughly chew two tablets twenty minutes before meals.
- If you are caught short and need fast relief, Phillip's Milk of Magnesia is merely magnesium oxide, and does not contain the aluminum that Maalox, Mylanta, and Di-Gel contain, and which is implicated in Parkinson's and Alzheimer's. It may have a laxative effect as well, but you should probably be hurrying things along anyway if you have overindulged.
- Baking soda in a glass of water (which is what Alka-Seltzer is without the fizz) can sop up or neutralize excess acid and alcohol.
- If caught with indigestion at a restaurant, bar, airport, or ship, try a teaspoon of Angostura Bitters in mineral water.
- Also, if digestive enzymes have not worked in the past or made you worse, you may really have too much acid. Remembering that the solution to pollution is dilution, you could drink a trial of a couple of glasses of spring water with meals to dilute the acid. This works better with food allergy or the Candida diet of whole foods and Rhizinate.
- Kudzu tea (in health food stores or catalogs in the Resource Guide) is a soothing root that is tasteless. One tablespoon of kudzu root powder mixed with any organic Chinese or Japanese green tea or macrobiotic kukicha tea with a few drops of shoyu sauce and pieces of half an umeboshi plum is soothing. This type of remedy works best for folks who already eat the macrobiotic way.

Achalasia

Achalasia actually means incomplete relaxation and emptying of the gastroesophageal area. It is sometimes misdiagnosed as reflux, hiatus hernia, or GERD, because it can present with any of their exact symptoms as given above.

Having a different origin, achalasia is actually caused by degeneration of the nerves in the esophagus, called the myenteric plexus. Because it causes the same heartburn symptoms as reflux and gastritis, it can be indistinguishable without a manometric (pressure) study. To perform this study a tube is inserted into the stomach to measure the pressure in the stomach and esophagus.

This is a diagnosis of elimination. In other words when all else fails, you may decide to get a manometric study to determine if achalasia or damaged esophageal nerves is the cause of your symptoms, for not much else distinguishes it from heartburn or other causes that I have described. Luckily, the treatments for either gastritis or GERD often solve the problem. But if they fail, use the Nutrition Protocol* to facilitate healing of the deteriorated nerves and check for diabetes as the cause of nerve damage.

Ulcer, Peptic Ulcer, Duodenal Ulcer, Gastric Ulcer

Even ulcers can be sneaky, fooling you into thinking you have something else. They can present as gastritis with just nausea and vomiting or indigestion with that unmistakable feeling of fullness, queasiness, and burning. But their usual symptom is intense burning along with a different type of pain that lets you know something is definitely wrong.

Sometimes the pain can feel as though it originates mid-back, directly behind the pit of the stomach. If you have such pain, be sure to have your doctor check for cancer of the pancreas. Never let ulcers go undiagnosed, for they can bleed and perforate the stomach, creating a hole that leads into the peritoneal (gut) cavity or abdomen. This is dangerous: You could bleed to death or get a nasty infection from the stomach contents that spill into the gut cavity. Such an infection is very difficult to treat and can cause problems for years to come—or can even be fatal. Problems can range from recurrent infections to adhesions or scar tissue that binds the intestine and inhibits its normal muscular contractions that propel food through the gut.

In regard to ulcers, it's also paramount that you do not have *H. pylori* because this can eventually cause stomach cancer. To know where you stand here, have your doctor measure the titer (amount of antibody in your blood) on two separate occasions. The test will tell you whether your infection is current or not.

In the meantime, while awaiting the results of the two titers, do a therapeutic trial of Pepto-Bismol, taking two to four caplets (or two tablespoons of the liquid) three to four times a day, one dose being before bed, for two weeks. You can then do another titer to determine whether your less-toxic treatment was a success. For any positive blood test, regardless of how low it is, be sure to have a follow-up test in a year. You need to follow up because of the high recurrence rate (even with no symptoms!) and the high association with future stomach cancer. Also, taking Helicobactrin, two capsules between meals two to three times a day (Ecologic Formulas) provides special mucin and other factors that promote healing.

Assuming the problem is not *H. pylori,* or it was and you got rid of it but still have symptoms, rule out food allergy next, and then Candida overgrowth (especially after any antibiotic treatment).

All the protocols for gastritis apply. In fact, because you know how you feel and how your medical history reflects that best, you are the one to decide which therapy might provide the quickest results. For example, if you know you have not taken many antibiotics and you have never had food allergies, then you would be more likely to check out the chances of having *H. pylori.*

As always, when the more common items fail to give you the answer, be sure you have had mineral and fatty acid analyses to learn why you are not healing. Low zinc, omega-3 fatty acids or vitamin A levels are common causes of delayed healing. Perfect for the last two is one daily teaspoon of Norwegian Cod Liver Oil (Carlson's).

Drinking juice three to four times a day to bathe the ulcer in phytochemicals that aid healing can also hurry healing. Juice combinations of carrot, celery, beet, cabbage, and cucumber work best.

Where do ulcers most commonly occur?—in the stomach and the duodenum, the tube that connects the stomach and the small intestine. Since the stomach is normally a high-acid environment, neutralizing the acid by alkalinizing the stomach often does no good. In fact, studies have shown it causes a rebound hypersecretion of even more acid, as though the stomach knows it has a deficient supply of acid and so overcompensates by secreting even more.

Duodenal ulcers, however, are just the opposite. They are normally bathed in the alkaline secretions of the pancreas. Nevertheless, to use antacids may provoke a heightened rebound secretion of acid from the stomach. This is one more reason why it is preferable to find the cause, whether *H. pylori,* hidden food allergy, or fungal infection, rather than relying solely on TV or prescribed medications for the symptoms mentioned.

Gallbladder Disease

There is no mistaking a gallbladder attack. It can present as a variety of symptoms, and even mimic a heart attack. But its reoccurence with fatty meals is the key. Most folks can turn the symptoms on and off like flicking a switch by eating fatty meals; cream sauces, sausages, candies, cheesecake, french fries, and juicy hamburgers are a few of the culprits.

Classic symptoms are tremendous pain and bloating, either up under the right ribs or in the pit of the stomach. Sometimes the pain feels more like it's in the right shoulder, because a branch of one of the nerves that supply the gallbladder runs up there.

The solution is a very low-fat diet with no fake fats or fat substitutes, and no processed foods. Drink plenty of liquids between meals, adding up to at least two eight-ounce glasses of spring water four to eight times a day.

Gallstones are the result of faulty chemistry prompted by the foods you eat, the liquids you drink, the cigarettes you smoke, and other factors in your diet and lifestyle. For example, every cigarette uses up about 100 milligrams of vitamin C that could have been used to beef up the immune system to kill bugs lurking in the gallbladder, bugs that can trigger gallstone formation. Vitamin C also inhibits stones from forming by yet another mechanism—by acidifying gallbladder contents. If the contents of the gallbladder are kept liquid and flowing, infection cannot build up and create the onionlike layering of cholesterol around accumulated sludge and bugs. As more cholesterol and other substances are laid down the stones grow bigger.

Every glass of soda flushes out priceless nutrients that should have been used to neutralize free radicals from our everyday chemicals. Instead, these wild electrons go on to transform gallbladder fats and sticky sludge into rocky cholesterol balls.

Abnormal or unnatural fats containing trans fatty acids are particularly able to trigger stone formation, just as they promote abnormal calcifications in coronary (heart) blood vessels. The worst foods having the highest trans fatty acid levels include margarines, hydrogenated polyunsaturated vegetable oils, and shortening. The most ubiquitous culprit is innocently labeled as soy (or soybean) oil. Do not eat any of these.

Let's look at some of the many dietary and metabolic errors (some or all) that contribute to the formation of gallstones:

- pulling calcium out of bones by smoking;
- a poor diet of sodas and processed foods;
- low vitamin and mineral levels so that calcium cannot be held in the bone;
- low acid or vitamin C level in the stomach, allowing growth of organisms in the gut and gallbladder;
- poor fluid intake, leaving gallbladder sludge to thicken and form stones;
- high-fat diets, especially of hydrogenated (soy or cottonseed) oils with trans fatty acids;
- high-cholesterol diet;
- food and chemical sensitivities; and more.

Some folks can do the gallbladder flush* and hoe out the gallbladder without surgery. Others are equally successful with a low-fat diet over several years, macrobiotic being the best here. A hypoallergenic diet, correcting nutrient deficiencies, or correcting digestive enzyme deficiencies can reverse gallbladder disease as well.

If I had gallstones or gallbladder disease, I would take the macrobiotic diet route, with which many have also reversed end-stage cancers after medicine had given up on them. It is a wholesome diet of whole grains, greens and beans, seeds and weeds, roots and fruits, and no processed foods. Although the macrobiotic diet requires a commitment both to learn and to follow it, it is well worth the effort, especially if you are threatened with surgery.

Folks not willing to go that extra mile can be successful merely by reading all labels on foods and avoiding a daily total of fats over ten to twenty grams. The problem with not eating the large variety of foods that a macrobiotic diet provides, is that such folks frequently end up with nutrient deficiencies within a few years and other diseases as a result. That's why a popular quick fix in this potentially serious problem is surgical.

Remember, an important first step for all regimens involves the elimination or vast reduction of sugars in cakes, cookies, candies, and other processed foods. X rays have confirmed that the bile was much thicker (more concentrated sludge) after six weeks of refined carbohydrates or flour and sugar products (Thornton). Nor should you neglect to identify possible hidden food allergies. In one study, folks had marked improvement in gallbladder symptoms within three to five days of following a diet that eliminated common allergens, including such trigger foods as egg, pork, and onion (Breneman).

I would also do a daily detox enema*, which empties the gallbladder so well as to remain invisible both on standard and sensitive ultrafast, X rays.

Abdominal Pain, Gas, Cramps, Diarrhea, Indigestion, IBS, IBD

Irritable bowel syndrome (IBS) is a catchall medical diagnosis. When there is no physical evidence to explain any gut symptom you can think of (like ulcer or cancer), doctors turn to IBS. In its way it's comforting to know that you have something, even if it presents with a variety of symptoms. With IBS, however, you can have any of the symptoms we have talked about for all the conditions above, and the discomfort can be anywhere in the abdomen.

Should you want to know more, then forge ahead. First priority, however, is to rule out food allergies, then Candida. Of course, by following the

Candida diet, you will also avoid many junk foods and wheat, sugar, and dairy products at the same time. Thus for many folks, the Candida diet is all they need since they thereby avoid the most common food antigens. In this sense the Candida diet is doubly healing with half the effort.

If these protocols fail, you'll probably want to know what uninvited guests might be living in your gut. Or before you spend the money on testing, you may want to try one of the many combination herbal protocols that cleanse the gut of undesirable bugs. One of my favorites is Paragard (Tyler): Take two to three capsules, two to three times a day for a month, between meals.

By all means, do the probiotic protocol and restore the good bugs or flora that give the bad bugs or flora competition as well as boost the power of the gut's immune system. Vital-Plex (Klaire) or Enterogenic Concentrate (Tyler) are a good start here; use either one to two capsules one to four times a day—as many as you can tolerate without excess gas. Use probiotics between meals to lessen the chance of stomach acid destroying the good bugs.

Now you can appreciate how over-the-counter drugs advertised as good for intestinal gas, for example, become self-perpetuating products. By relieving gas symptoms temporarily, these drugs also set the stage for more gas later on. As they do nothing to kill the bad bugs that cause gas, you can never be cured by taking them. Gas can be caused by only two things: by eating foods that you do not have enough enzymes to digest properly or by the presence of bad bugs in higher numbers than can be tolerated, or which do not belong in the gut at all.

Should you have diarrhea, I suggest here that you let it run its course unless you are in dire straits and growing weak and dehydrated. Try to identify what your body wants so valiantly to get rid of and help it along. For example, if you went out for dinner and had diarrhea by the next day, you obviously ate something that's bad for your body. So why would you want to prevent yourself from excreting it with an antidiarrheal medication?

Many people have visited a foreign country and used diarrhea-inhibiting medications for the relentless diarrhea of tourists *(tourista),* only to make matters worse. By the time they returned home, having kept this nasty bug hostage in their gut for days, it had grown into threatening numbers. Then it was all the more difficult to eradicate and required powerful medications with nasty side effects. And all because they did not listen to the wisdom of the body and get rid of the bug as nature intended.

There is one product though, designed by biochemist Dr. Jeffrey Bland, which does help to heal the gut when it's attacked by a toxic substance, whether that comes from a particular food or not: UltraInflamX. With

UltraInflamX, Dr. Bland covers as many areas of the irritable bowel as possible, combining the low allergy-generating potential of a vegeterian powder with vitamins, minerals, and other nutrients. In fact, UltraInflamX is designed to help the gut heal itself by revving up its capacity to detoxify while turning down the inflammatory response (Satoskar). Begin with half a scoop dissolved in water or juice twice a day. A patient booklet accompanies UltraInflamX and it is readily available from HealthComm International, the company that produces it.

Remember: the cause for IBS in most folks is food allergy, Candida overgrowth, or both conditions at once. And you should now be a pro at treating these.

Constipation

Normally you should have one to two well-formed bowel movements a day. Anything less than that will eventually deteriorate your health by initiating an avalanche of seemingly unrelated symptoms as toxins overwhelm your organs. Constipation also includes difficult-to-pass stools that require straining. Straining, of course, can create hemorrhoids, varicose veins, diverticuli, and even the weakening and ballooning of brain vessels, eventually leading to stroke.

I feel that it is impossible to be truly healthy as long as you are constipated. If, by chance, someone is constipated but feels great otherwise, I would not anticipate this wellness to continue. There are many fine sources of fiber to correct constipation quickly. But you need to identify the cause, which may be any of the causes of IBS.

Constipation is usually caused by a combination of things:

- bad bugs in the gut putting out toxins that intoxicate or nearly paralyze normal nerve-to-muscle function.
- food allergies that inflame the gut lining, impairing function as well.
- nutrient deficiencies, especially magnesium, which is very common in over a third of the population.
- poor selection of processed, overcooked fiber-poor foods. Just avoiding all processed foods, especially cheese, bread, sugar, and alcohol, and having at least one to two shredded raw vegetable salads a day and buck-flower cereal each morning (equal parts of raw buckwheat grauts and sunflower seeds soaked overnight, to which you may add any fruits or liquids in the morning) can solve constipation. The more fiber in the colon in the form of raw fruits and vegetables, whole grains, beans, seeds and nuts, the more water that is pulled into the

stool to bulk it up. This stimulates peristalsis, the muscular contractions that propel stool out of the colon.

One of the most simultaneously healthful and effective therapies for constipation is the vitamin C cocktail (also called the vitamin C flush—see Chapter 5) taken to bowel tolerance.

Depending on your allergies, there are a variety of fine fiber products as well. **But remember:** you must drink at least two large glasses of good water when taking them. These sources of water-attracting fiber work by pulling water into the stool to make it more liquid.

Fiber-Cleansing Protocols

Use any of the products listed below. They all have unique combinations of ingredients and are all effective products. Because of the wide array of herbals used, they add bulk to the stool, soften the contents of the stool, stimulate the muscular contractions of the gut (peristalsis), and detoxify gut contents. Product differences here also depend on the differences among people, their biochemical individuality, which includes their allergies.

- Herbal Laxative (Thorne) contains blue flag, rhubarb, buckthorn, senna, and cascara. Take one to two capsules before bed with two large glasses of water.
- UltraFiber (HealthComm) contains cellulose, beet, barley, apple, rice, and tocotrienols. Take two scoops one to two times a day.
- Flax Fiber (Jarrow) contains organic flaxseed powder. Use one to two tablespoons in two large glasses of water a day.
- Nutra-Flax 1000 (Pure Encapsulations) contains organic flaxseed powder. Take three to twelve capsules a day, in any way you like.
- Fiber-Plex (Klaire) is made from apple, oat, orange, acacia, cellulose, and sodium choleate. Take one to three tablets with abundant water three times a day, a half hour before meals.
- Fiber Formula (Tyler) contains psyllium, oat, bentonite, bromelain and other enzymes, herbs, vitamins, and is the only fiber formula I know with probiotics as well. Use one-half to one tablespoon in a large glass of water, two to three times a day.
- FiberPlus (PhytoPharmica) contains psyllium, grapefruit pectin, oat, carrot, prune, and beet fiber, as well as FOS and many healing herbs, including aloe vera, marshmallow, chamomile, goldenseal, berberine. Take two to six capsules twice a day.
- Laxatol (PhytoPharmica) contains aloe vera extract plus rhubarb, prune, and ginger extracts. Take one to two capsules before bed.

- Nature's Pure Body Program (Pure Body Institute). See Chapter 5 for directions.

As with any product for constipation, the biggest concern is for an obstruction. Scar tissue (adhesions) from former abdominal surgery, radiation, tumor, or infection can slowly grow and wrap around segments of bowel, dangerously strangling them. Or a segment of bowel can twist and strangle itself (called a volvulus, and diagnosed on X ray). In either case, if the strangulation becomes complete, putting anything else into the gut can cause it to rupture or explode—a possibly fatal event. So never keep taking laxatives if they do not work within a few days, if you have a fever, or if the pain worsens. See a physician.

Hemorrhoids

You know you have hemorrhoids if you notice a very soft lump outside the rectum, or any itching, bleeding (bright red blood, seen usually on any toilet paper you use or on the outside of the stool), or unmistakable rectal pain, especially when sitting or walking.

Hemorrhoids, of course, are merely rectal blood vessels that are dilated from increased pressure that has stretched them beyond their capacity to return to normal size. Predominating causes include constipation, obesity, pregnancy, heavy lifting, and prolonged sitting, as well as deficiencies of copper, manganese, sulfur, fatty acids like the omega-3 oil DHA, and other nutrients that weaken blood-vessel walls.

Passing a big constipated stool past swollen, bleeding hemorrhoids can be exceedingly painful. In the heat of the moment, many folks have wondered if they would survive the pain. The good news is that you can heal such hemorrhoids without surgery. And healing begins with an enema.

First, get a small, fine tip to attach to your enema bag. If you cannot find a urinary catheter in a medical supply store, ask your doctor to write a prescription for a #28 French catheter. Lubricate it well with olive oil before inserting it among those delicate and painful hemorrhoids.

Do the detox enema (with your fine tip attached to the bag) at least once or twice a day, to keep the volume of stool small and liquid. You don't want to pass any big stools that will open the healing rectal tears or cause the hemorrhoids to bleed. You want to rest all the damaged tissues while they heal for a few weeks. Use a stool softener—a fiber product designed for constipation—every day as well to keep the stools nice and mushy.

If your butt is very painful, you can sit with it in a big salad bowl filled with one teaspoon sea salt for every cup of tepid filtered water or you can add two to three cups of Epsom salts (grocery or drug store) to your bath water. Once you get past the first few painful days of acute hemorrhoids, you will never let yourself get that constipated again.

Diverticulitis

Diverticulitis is a common result of IBS syndrome, which can also present as pain in a specific area of the gut. When that happens, folks sometimes worry that a cancer may be present. You'll suspect it's not cancer, though, if symptoms appear only when eating certain high-roughage foods like seeds, berries with seeds, and nuts.

Diverticuli are like tiny pouches or appendices that stick or balloon out from the gut wall from years of constipation. Once they emerge high-roughage foods can lodge within them, causing irritation, inflammation, or worse yet, infection.

If you have diverticulitis, you'll quickly learn what foods trigger it, what foods to avoid, and how to prepare the other foods you normally eat. It's best to stick to well-cooked, soft, and easy-to-digest foods until the symptoms (and pain) have subsided.

For the sake of good health, gradually introduce more natural fiber from raw fruits and vegetables into your diet. If you can't tolerate such foods, then try one of the fiber formulas just described. Start with the lowest dose and move up ever so slowly, being careful not to trigger irritation and symptoms. You must get your stools moving at least once a day or those diverticuli become cesspools just begging to get massively infected.

If the fiber formula solutions are too irritating even at low doses, start with a milder laxative like Laxatol. Also, any herbs that have antibacterial properties are helpful in discouraging infection, including Paragard, Oil of Oregano, and garlic compounds.

Another very helpful therapy is the detox enema, especially when the "tics" (as they are referred to in the trade) get inflamed and painful. In addition, you'll want to do the nutrient protocol to improve their ability to heal and avoid perforation.

Crohn's Disease, Blood and Mucus Colitis, Ulcerative Colitis, Regional Enteritis, Regional Ileitis

Folks with Crohn's disease, blood and mucus colitis, ulcerative colitis, regional enteritis, and regional ileitis are among the sickest with bowel disease. They have incredible pain and usually blood and or mucus, as well as frequent diarrhea. They are in misery. Even if they present with just diarrhea, it occurs after every meal and often a half dozen more times between meals as well.

Diagnoses for these conditions should be taken seriously; they are the most difficult to heal because they invariably involve the largest number of factors contributing to total load. In addition, they can be life threatening, causing bleeding and weight loss, or requiring transfusion or surgery. Folks with such conditions usually have been hospitalized several times and take many prescribed medications. They all need personalized, professional help. Nonetheless, having stumbled onto what caused the condition, many folks are able to keep it from intensifying, and many clear completely.

Dan had his first bout of bloody mucus and painful diarrhea in college. He had a standard work-up while hospitalized, and he required two transfusions. Once out of the hospital, he found it convenient to take the four medications his doctor prescribed, which allowed him the relative freedom he needed to carry on his sales business. As it was, he knew the location of the nearest bathroom at every call.

Within a few years, after several more emergency hospitalizations for flare-ups, his gastroenterologists were threatening a bowel resection. One area of the colon was particularly damaged and the source of most of the bleeding. His doctors felt that surgically removing the several feet of intestine comprising that area would free him from his symptoms. All well and good but, because the problematic area was low down in the colon, he would have to wear a colostomy bag attached to his stomach for the rest of his life.

Dan finally came to me when he decided to explore other options. First we looked for what might be growing in the colon, then for hidden food allergies, as well as nutrient and digestive enzyme deficiencies. Within six months, his colon had calmed down enough to require no medications. Six years later, Dan has not been hospitalized again and he has learned how to look for the cause if he starts to experience even the slightest amount of former symptoms.

It is imperative that the victim of serious colitis carefully rule out food allergies. Many do much better with additional testing and the administration of injections for allergies to foods as well as pollen, dust, and molds, for their guts are a target organ for what they eat, drink, and breathe. This is especially important if there is a current or previous history of allergies, recurrent respiratory infections, sore throats or sinusitis, bronchitis, asthma, or eczema.

In such cases, every gut test must be done; no stone can be left unturned. (See Chapter 7.) I would also empirically treat for yeast even if it were not found, since it makes a dramatic difference in so many despite a negative test. It is especially important, if there is a long history of use of antibiotics for acne, prostatitis, cystitis, recurrent sinusitis or bronchitis, steroids, or other hormones.

In addition, on stool assay you will usually find an assortment of nasty bugs and parasites in the gut. The report tells of many antibiotics to which these bugs are sensitive. Antibiotics though are the last thing we want to use. Fortunately, there is an herb called artemisia that many of these bacteria and protozoa are sensitive to. In fact, artemisia is so potent that it has been used to kill malaria, and you'll recall it was one of the herbs in Paragard. The highest dose I have found is 500 milligrams of *Artemisia annua* in Artecin (Thorne/ARG). Take at least a two-to-four-week trial of two capsules three times a day, then repeat the culture to check its effectiveness.

For those who have lost weight, there is no substitute for ruling out gluten enteropathy (celiac disease—see Chapter 2) followed by a six-month therapeutic trial, regardless of results. This means strict avoidance of the slightest bit of wheat, oats, rye, or barley. To accomplish this, you need to eat very simple, unadorned foods, in a form as close to nature (unprocessed) as possible. Imperative is the avoidance of foods with a list of ingredients that you cannot thoroughly translate, or foods that you do not know the precise recipe for, and any possible substitutions that could have been made.

In fact with serious cases, when in doubt, and especialy when eating out, a simple rule applies: Folks are better off making their own food for dining out with friends, and, yes, eating it at the restaurant. After all, camaraderie is as much or more a reason for eating out with friends as the food. Moreover, most folks can make as good or better, and certainly more nutritious, meals at home than any restaurant. In fulfilling the terms of the celiac diet with the precision needed for serious disease, it is imperative to be very cognizant of all gluten sources.

For example, some folks new to the disorder and champing at the bit for a bread substitute will search out breads that are wheat-free, whether to eat at home or in a restaurant. But I have never been to a grain mill that did not have a cloud of wheat dust in the air. That means that microscopic wheat antigen contaminates all their products. It is foolhardy to risk a six-month flare-up of malabsorption over one piece of bread. Include dairy-free and disaccharide-free diets here as well. (See Chapter 2.)

Sometimes the gut is so damaged that it needs to rest. If you had a broken leg, you would not be out dancing every night. Yet we think nothing of asking the gut to carry on its thrice daily activity of digesting food. Total hyperalimentation (feeding nutrients and food substitutes by vein) allows the gut to rest.

I know where I would go should my gut be so damaged: the Environmental Health Center in Dallas under the direction of Dr. William J. Rea (address in Resources section). Dr. Rea has a unique dual specialty certification in surgery and environmental medicine, with his expertise extending to nutritional biochemistry and toxicology. He has written a four-volume textbook for physicians (*Chemical Sensitivity*, Boca Raton, FL, CRC Press, 1990–1998) and his accomplishments do not end there, for he has successfully treated more severely environmentally damaged, undiagnosable, and untreatable individuals than anyone I personally know or know of.

If you cannot afford to go to Dallas, consider doing the nutrition protocol III, supplying nutrients via the rectal route to allow the gut some healing time. Use L-glutamine, butyric acid, and vitamin C by retention enema, and you could even add Nutricillin and Sialex by oral or rectal route. Remember to keep L-glutamine separate from the rest.

If you want to try to nourish the body through a damaged gut without hyperalimentation, you will need foods that are already predigested, in a ready-to-use form for the body. By starting with more readily assimilable foods, you are effectively relieving the gut of some of its work. A product called Sea Cure (made by Proper Nutrition) does this quite well. Hydrolyzed from deep ocean white fish, it contains 85 percent protein in a form ready to use by the damaged gut. In addition, Sea Cure provides a natural source of omega-3 fatty acids necessary for healing the gut. Take two to four capsules, two to three times a day before meals.

An additional option that many folks do exceedingly well with, for use alone or in combination with Sea Cure, is Ultra Clear (made by HealthComm). Use one to two scoops two to three times a day in a large glass of water. Ultra Clear contains nutrients to aid in healing the gut plus some hypoallergenic calories (rice antigen), thus giving the gut a rest.

If absorption is a problem, I recommend BottomsUp (ARG/ Nutricology), which is taken rectally. BottomsUp is one of several products that enables you to "feed" your system nutrients by the rectal route, as I will explain later on in this chapter.

It is also important to take L-glutamine, 500 to 2000 milligrams two to four times a day in powder form preferably, but which may be taken in capsule form if necessary. Be sure to take it two hours before or after meals, as digestive acidity destroys it.

Of equal importance is getting enough butyric acid, through one to three daily retention enemas (Tyler—described later), or Cal-Mag Butyrate capsules (Ecologic Formulas), one to six taken after meals. Butyric acid is particularly necessary for the healing gut and, in fact, has caused some gut cancers to redifferentiate, or return to normal cells once again.

Natural Antibiotics Protocol

Folks with serious colitis frequently have major infections in the gut that actually instigated their colitis. Often those infections are still lurking, causing the colitis to persist, however mysteriously it may seem to do so. For this you need antibiotic power that will not stimulate Candida overgrowth, as all artificial antibiotics do. Nutricillin (made by Ecologic Formulas) contains lactoferrin and olive leaf extract, both of which are natural products with strong antibactrial, antiviral, and antifungal properties (Samaranayaki, Hasegawa, Okutomi, Ellison, Tranter, Walker, Juven). In fact, Nutricillin is an excellent product for folks with resistant Candida overgrowth that does not respond to other nutrients (Bellamy). Its ingredients have a record not only for inhibiting colon cancer (Oguchi), but also for protecting the gut against radiation colitis (Shimmura). Take one to three capsules two to three times a day.

Nutricillin contains, in addition to 60 milligrams Lactoferrin and 50 milligrams of olive leaf extract, 150 milligrams of colostrum and 60,000 units of lysozyme. If you want to evaluate the effect of higher doses of the antimicrobial agent lactoferrin alone, it is available as a singular substance as Lactoferrin 100 milligrams (Ecologic Formulas) or with colostrum in 350 milligram capsules as Laktferrin (ARG/Nutricology). Take one to three before going to bed. In addition, all 600 milligrams of thymic extract in the form of lyphoactivated thymic peptides (LTP) (Ecologic Formulas), taking two to four a day to boost infection fighting capacity.

Special Intestinal Support Protocol

Studies on serious colitis show a marked deficiency of a certain type of mucin, a thick mucus layer designed to protect the gut wall from invasion and injury. Sialic acid (neuraminic acid) is not only physically protective, but also an antioxidant to boot (Rhodes, Forstner) and can be restored with Sialex (Ecologic Formulas); take one to three after meals. And don't forget, these potent therapies for colitis can also be used for resistant cases of IBS, leaky gut, and Candida overgrowth. Sialex can be combined with LTP, or with Nutricillin or Lactoferrin and UltraInflamX.

The fact is that the colitis victim needs anything he or she can tolerate that helps to improve the integrity of his or her severely damaged gut. Because the breakdown product of the damaged gut overloads the liver and in turn intoxicates the gut even more, take herbs to strengthen the liver like Thisilibin (Bio-Tech) or Hepagen (Ecologic Formulas). Each contains silymarin, a potent herb to rescue the liver. Take two to four a day.

Before moving on to the next gut malady, let's look at just one of the prescription drugs for colitis to remind you of how drug-driven medicine nearly always guarantees that the sick will get sicker, while cause-concerned medicine pushes you closer to healing. As you must now realize, the more serious the condition, often the more serious the side effects of prescribed medications, justified presumably because there is no alternative (or so doctors lead you to believe).

Sulfasalazine, also known by the trade name Azulfidine and (its new cousin) Asacol, is a time-honored drug. Side effects include kidney or lung damage so severe it can be lethal, paralysis (Guillain-Barré syndrome), hepatitis, depression, vision problems, and even a low white blood cell count (leukopenia) and a decreased level of blood clotting cells (thrombocytopenia), both of which are particularly dangerous for someone already run-down by intestinal infection and bleeding.

Sulfasalizine is universally prescribed for most colitis patients, in the acute stage as well as "forever" with hopes of keeping them in remission. It is a glorified aspirin (NSAID) and sulfa drug rolled into one. By now you recognize that as a deadly duo guaranteed to make and maintain a leaky gut indefinitely. And that is one reason colitis patients rarely recover permanently: They are prescribed drugs that perpetuate the disease and, in fact, worsen it, methodically decreasing the chance for recovery.

Candida, Intestinal Dysbiosis, Parasites

As you must know by now, you don't have to have any gut symptoms to have the worst case of Candida-related syndrome going. The toxins released into the bloodstream by this bug can mimic fibromyalgia, chronic fatigue syndrome, chemical and food sensitivities, and many other conditions. Or if the Candida overgrowth has triggered LGS, you can suffer anything from mild gas and bloating to terrible cramps and diarrhea.

Whatever uninvited bugs are growing in the gut, you need to get rid of them or at least reduce their numbers. Candida is not abnormal in the gut, but it *is* abnormal when among the top ten organisms seen on a stool test. With over 500 bugs in the intestines to digest food, produce vitamins, and produce healing enzymes for the gut, Candida should not be a predominating bug, readily visible on a screening study.

So even if the test results show Candida to be at the lowest level reportable (one plus, or 1 +), do not consider that normal. Many doctors will tell folks not to worry, that 1+ is just a little bit of Candida and need not be treated. Unfortunately, that is like telling someone they are just a little bit pregnant or have just a little bit of cancer. As I have noted again and again, I find dramatic improvements in gut symptoms, not to mention other seemingly unrelated symptoms, whenever I treat a 1+ Candida level.

Intestinal dysbiosis from any other cause needs a CDSA and/or purged parasites test to identify the other unwanted intruders. Or if you cannot afford a test, a blind trial of Paragard or other broad spectrum herbals, like the Nature's Pure Body Program, may reduce unwanted intestinal bugs.

Cancer

Like many gut conditions, cancer can be a great imitator on its own. You need not have any symptoms at all in the early stages, and it can be found quite by accident. Or you can quickly go downhill with unmistakable bleeding, weight loss, and pain.

There are only two ways I have seen folks heal cancer, even when all that medicine has to offer them has failed. One way is the live food diet (described in my newsletter) where 80% of the diet is raw fruits, vegetables, nuts and seeds. The remainder of the diet consists of soaked or sprouted grains, seeds and beans, and a small amount of minimally cooked food. The superior and most documented healing treatment involves the macrobiotic diet, which is generally much better tolerated by those with any intestinal symptoms. Refer to my books, *You Are What You Ate, The Cure Is in the Kitchen,* and *Wellness Against All Odds,* for more information on macrobiotics. My book catalog also mentions other autobiographical books on successes in healing cancer as well as further treatment plans. (See the Resource Guide.)

A Quick Summary of Treatments

Remember, for any condition you may need to follow only one or two protocols to find the cause or causes and get relief. Only those with more severe or resistant cases will need to follow many protocols. The odds are in your favor. As always, I assume that you have had a GI medical evaluation, nothing was found, and cancers were ruled out.

If This Is Overwhelming . . .

Although I have not given you the entire gamut of causes of and cures for gut symptoms, your head may be reeling with all the new knowledge you now possess. You and I both know that finding the cause is key to the cure, whether it be *H. pylori,* Candida overgrowth, food allergies, other bugs, poor eating habits, or something else. But in the meantime, you need some symptomatic relief.

I've outlined a few quick fixes for common symptoms, but don't be surprised if some actually cure the problem, for that is one of the "side effects" of a natural approach. For example, instead of using H2-blockers for heartburn, you may find you need to enhance, rather than inhibit, natural function. Digestive enzymes, like Similase or Biogest, may clear up the symptom once and for all if you have become deficient in making enough

Table 12. Summary of Treatments

Condition	For diagnosis and/or treatment	Laboratory test
Mouth sores, canker sores Aphthous stomatitis analysis)	Diagnostic diet for food Allergies DGL/Rhizinate protocol Kyolic/Kyo-Greens Tea tree oil Pure Body Program WaterOz Silver Vitamin C flush Detox enema	Mineral analysis EFA (essential fatty acid)
Halitosis	Rule out infection of sinuses, teeth, gums. food allergy Lack of chewing Candida Digestive enzymes Probiotics	CDSA
Nausea, vomiting	Rule out pregnancy, brain tumor, ear infection, chemical toxicity or sensitivity, medication sensitivity. diagnostic diet GingerMax	CDSA
Hiatus hernia, GERD, acid heartburn, reflux esophagitis	Smaller meals, elevation of head of bed, nocturnal aloe vera Parasympathetic protocol Rhizinate or Gastro-Relief Food allergy (diagnostic diet) H. pylori protocol Candida protocol	*H. pylori* antibodies CDSA Candida antibodies
Gastritis, heartburn esophagitis, NUD, dyspepsia, acid indigestion, achalasia	Smaller more peaceful meals, chewing Parasympathetic protocol Rhizinate Digestive enzymes Diagnostic diet Candida protocol *H. pylori* protocol Aloe vera Milk of magnesia 8 oz water every hour while awake	H. pylori antibodies CDSA Candida antibodies

Table 12. Summary of Treatments *(cont.)*

Condition	For diagnosis and/or treatment	Laboratory test
Achalasia	Nutrition protocol	Minerals EFA CDSA Vitamins
Ulcer, peptic ulcer, duodenal ulcer, gastric ulcer	H. pylori protocol Candida protocol Gastritis protocols Juicing	H. pylori antibodies Mineral EFA (fatty acids) L-glutamine
Gallbladder disease	Low-fat diet 8 oz water 6–12 times a day Apple cider vinegar Digestive enzymes Diagnostic diet Vitamin C flush Gallbladder flush	Minerals EFA
Spastic colitis, gas, cramps, intermittent diarrhea and/or constipation, indigestion, IBS, short but frequent bouts of abdominal pain	Food allergies (diagnostic diet) Candida Fiber from natural laxatives Pure Body Protcol Probiotics UltraInflamX L-glutamine Paragard Celiac diet	celiac antibodies CDSA Purged parasites Leaky gut test Organic acids Food allergy panel Minerals EFA CDSA Thyroid antibodies
Hemorrhoids, constipation, and diverticulitis	Fiber from whole wheat Water Probiotics Candida Food allergies (diagnostic diet) Vitamin C flush Natural laxatives	Minerals EFA CDSA Thyroid autoantibodies
Crohn's disease, blood and mucus colitis, ulcerative colitis, regional enteritis, regional ileitis	Diagnostic diet Food and environmental (chemical, dust, pollen, mold allergies) Candida Nutrient protocol	CDSA Purged parasites Leaky gut test 7-Day Candida Culture Mineral assays Fatty-acid assay

Table 12. Summary of Treatments *(cont.)*		
Condition	For diagnosis and/or treatment	Laboratory test
Crohn's disease, blood and mucus colitis, ulcerative colitis, regional enteritis, regional ileitis	Celiac diet Hyperalimentation or rectal route protocol Sialex Butyrate Nutricillin, Lactoferrin LTP Hepagen or Thisilibin	Vitamin assay Celiac antibodies (anti-gluten)
Candida, intestinal dysbiosis, parasites	Candida diet Paragard Candida antibodies Artecin or Citramesia	CDSA 7-Day Candida Culture Purged parasites Organic acids
Cancer	See text	Full workup

by yourself or are eating more wild food combinations than your digestive capability can meet.

Likewise, instead of enhancing your chances of getting Parkinson's disease, paralysis, or Alzheimer's disease by taking aluminum-containing antacids (Perl, Weberg, Bolla), it makes infinitely more sense to treat your ulcer with four cups (one liter or quart total) of freshly squeezed cabbage juice a day. Studies show it stopped ulcer pain within two to five days, and showed healing on X rays within an average of eleven days (Cheney). Because very few could tolerate this alone, use one part each of celery and carrots to every two to four parts cabbage.

Similarly, since IBS can so often be caused by overgrowth of uninvited gut bugs, giving them some competition from probiotics like VitalPlex or KyoDophilus can discourage their growth. There are also numerous items that discourage the growth of bugs, and are useful not only for immediate but often permanent relief of IBS or chronic diarrhea symptoms. For example, Candimyacin (PhytoPharmica) contains oregano oil as well as peppermint oil, both of which relieve IBS symptoms (Rees, Somerville).

Containing the immune-stimulating herb goldenseal plus another oil with antimicrobial properties, thyme oil, the dose is one to two capsules between meals.

Don't lose sight of the fact that if symptoms recur, you want to persist until you find the curable cause. It could be as simple as folks who cleared up chronic diarrhea with folic acid, which recurred when the supplementation was stopped (Carruthers).

As you don't need all these things in your nonmedicine chest, pick out a few based on your most common symptoms, so you are prepared for emergencies with natural solutions. How do you now spell relief? R-h-i-z-i-n-a-t-e.

The Rest of the Protocols

Now for the other protocols that you may want to refer to that were not described in the previous chapters.

Digestive Enzymes

If I didn't know better, I'd think we were on an intentionally self-destructive path for the pancreas. Look at all we do that tends to weaken and deplete our pancreatic reserves. Just the amount of sugar in the daily diet can stress it unmercifully. Sodas that don't contain the undesirable fake sugars sport anywhere from four to nine teaspoons of sugar, a very large amount that puts a huge demand on the pancreas for insulin. In addition, we eat many cooked and processed foods, which are really dead in terms of enzyme action. It is only the live or raw foods that contain the natural enzymes we need and that can replenish those the body makes for itself.

Add to that high amounts of dietary fats from french fries and other fried and fast foods, processed foods, and cheeses, butter, fatty meats, and delicious sweets, all of which put extra demand on pancreatic lipases and other enzymes. In addition, common deficiencies, such as zinc, can jeopardize pancreatic enzyme output. And even everyday home and office chemicals and pesticides can damage pancreatic enzyme function (Marsh).

Why all the fuss? Because pancreatic enzymes are not only a critical determinant of whether or not you get a cancer, but whether or not you conquer it. Indeed, pancreatic enzymes are a vital part of the body's police force for aberrant cancer cells that must be destroyed immediately. Without sufficient pancreatic enzymes, cancer cells, which we all have, can survive and grow. More important, once cancer has begun, pancreatic enzymes are vital for healing, especially in protocols that have been highly successful after everything that medicine had to offer has failed. Pancreatic enzymes

Table 13. Stock Your Nonmedicine Chest With These for a Quick Fix

Symptom	TV remedy	Natural remedy
Heartburn or indigestion	antacids, H2-blockers	Gastro-Relief (Rhizinate with calcium carbonate, so do not use with additional Rhizinate); Aloe vera gel or caps Rhizinate or Gastro-Relief; Similase or Biogest
Ulcer pain	antacids, H2-blockers, Prilosec	Gastro-Relief, Rhizinate, or Gastramet; Cabbage juice (sorry, it must be freshly juiced) or Gastramet; L-glutamine
IBS	Antacids, H2-blockers, Prilosec, antibiotics	Digestive enzymes, like Similase, Pancreatin, Biogest; L-glutamine ParaGard; Candimyacin; oil of oregano; tea tree oil; probiotics, like VitalPlex; Artesin; Nutricillin
Constipation	Laxatives	FiberPlex
Diarrhea	Anticholinergics, opiate derivatives, antibiotics	ParaGard; Candimyacin; oil of oregano; Cal-Mag Butyrate; probiotics, like VitalPlex or KyoDophilus; Kyolic; Garlinase; Artesin; Silver Mineral Water; tea tree oil; Pure Body Program
Nausea/vomiting	Anti-emetics	GingerMax
Preventing traveler's diarrhea (bring along in your suitcase)	Prescribed antibiotics or opiate antidiarrheals	Pepto-Bismol; Nutricillin; WaterOz Silver; Probiotics (like VitalPlex)

are the only natural substance we possess that dissolves off the protective armor of cancer cells that makes them invisible and thus invincible to the immune system.

Enzymes have other functions, like improving blood flow to difficult-to-reach areas with a poor blood supply, such as the bladder or prostate (Dittmar). That is why bladder or prostate conditions prompt doctors to prescribe prolonged and intensive doses of antibiotics. Pancreatic enzymes are aids here as well, ensuring the penetration of antibiotics into swollen, inflamed tissues that need them the most.

More important, pancreatic enzymes can imrove conditions such as lactase deficiency and celiac disease. For folks who simply need to boost their ability to tolerate dairy sugar, or lactose, the lactase contained in enzyme preparations is usually enough on its own to do the job. Similarly, some enzyme preparations have also enabled celiac disease patients to once again tolerate grains like wheat, which would otherwise set off toxic reactions (Phelan, McCarthy).

For folks who must avoid animal products, there are plant-derived enzymes available, like bromlain in pineapple or well-thought-out combinations of plant enzymes as in Similase. There are also options for those who, because of allergies, must avoid mold antigens common to plants and take enzymes from animal glands. Pancreatic enzymes are available as beef, lamb, or pork antigens, solo or in excellent combinations with other digestives.

Some folks, of course, just need more stomach acid for better digestion, in which case betaine hydrochloric acid (HCl) fits the bill. It can be taken alone or in combination with other enzymes. Always start with a low dose, one capsule before a meal, and build up slowly. If it feels too acidic or it burns, cut back to a dose that does not bother you. Don't be surprised if many other things improve when you take enzymes. When you start supplementing with enzymes, you can attain better digestion, heal your gut, have healthier nail and hair growth, and improved moods and energy.

Here are some of my favorite choices of enzymes for healing the gut. Each item is usually best tried on its own, although combinations can work later on. As with everything, your preference is a highly individual matter, thus the several excellent options below. You owe it to yourself to see if your indigestion isn't a lot better just with the addition of digestive enzymes.

If digestion improves, you should get your minerals tested; mineral deficiencies that have crept up over the years are a leading cause for deficient supplies of enzymes. For example, taking extra calcium to deter osteoporosis, can diminish your supply of zinc, which in turn decreases the amount of stomach acid and pancreatic enzymes you can make.

Here then are four of my favorite all-purpose enzyme combinations that help take over where deficient stomach, pancreatic, and other digestive enzymes leave off. You can try any one of them. You need not use a combination of enzymes. If you prefer to focus more specifically on whether you need stomach or pancreatic enzymes, or plant-based enzymes for allergic folks, I have provided these as well.

Multipurpose Digestive Enzymes

Similase (Tyler)
Similase contains thirteen different plant-based enzymes derived from vegetable sources, including lactase, sucrase, maltase, protease, amylase, lipase, and cellulase. In other words, it provides for the digestion of carbohydrates, protein, fats, fiber, dairy, sugars, and more. Take one to four capsules before each meal.

Panplex 2-Phase (Tyler)
Panplex 2-Phase contains betaine HCl; glutamic acid; pepsin, for phase one of stomach digestion; and pancreatin with amylase, protease, and lipase, plus ox bile, for phase two of gallbladder and pancreas digestion. Take one to two capsules with meals.

Biogest (Thorne)
Biogest contains betaine, pancreas, pepsin, ox bile, and glutamic acid (pork antigen). Take one to two capsules with meals.

Bio-Zyme (PhytoPharmica)
Bio-Zyme contains pancreas (protease, amylase, lipase), trypsin, papain, bromelain, amylase, lipase, lysozyme, and chymotrypsin. Take one to three capsules with meals.

Infla-Zyme Forte (American Biologics)
Infla-Zyme Forte contains pancreatinic bromelain, papain, trypsin, chymotrypsin, lipase, and more. Take one to three capsules with meals.

Stomach enzymes

Betaine HCl (Thorne)
Betaine HCl also contains pepsin. Take one to two capsules with meals. If the stomach feels too acidic or burns, obviously cut back on the dose, or stop taking it entirely.

Betaine HCl (Tyler)

Tyler's Betaine HCl also contains pepsin. Take one to two capsules with meals.

HCl and Pepsin (Carlson)

Take one to two capsules with meals, but cut back or stop taking it entirely if stomach feels too acidic

Digest III (Bio-Tech)

Take one to two capsules with meals.

Pancreatic enzymes

Dipan-9 (Thorne)

Dipan-9 contains high-potency, pure pancreatin, providing amylase, protease, and lipase. Take one to four capsules with meals.

Pancreas (Klaire)

Contains pure pancreas. Take one to four capsules with meals.

Pan 8 Supreme (Ecologic Formulas) contains pure pancreas. Take one to four capsules with meals.

Organic Pancreatin (ARG)

Organic Pancreatin comes as pork, lamb, or beef antigen. Take one to 6 capsules with meals as needed.

Bromelain

Bromelain Complex (PhytoPharmica)

Bromelain Complex also contains pantothenic acid and vitamin C. Take one to two capsules with meals.

Bromelain (Jarrow)

Bromelain, manufactured by Jarrow, is a natural, proteolytic enzyme (cysteine carboxypeptidase) derived from pineapple that has anti-inflammatory actions as well. It contains no soy, corn, wheat, yeast, or dairy antigens. Take one to four capsules with meals.

M.F. Bromelain (Thorne)

Take two capsules with meals.

Bromase (Bio-Tech)

Take one to two capsules with meals.

Detox Cocktail

Above and beyond the vitamin C flush, there is the detox cocktail, which revs up your ability to handle toxins of all sorts. If you drank too much alcohol the night before, feel like you are fighting a bad intestinal bug, or are suffering the side effects of an H2-blocker, the detox coktail is very useful for accelerating detoxification and for getting you back on track.

The formula is simple and the ingredients belong in your emergency drug cabinet. Add one heaping teaspoon of (Klaire's) Ultra Fine Ascorbic Acid Powder to one scoop and two 400 milligram capsules of (Tyler's) Recancostat in a large nine-ounce glass of good water. Follow by another eight-ounce glass of water. This may be repeated every two to six hours as needed. If you get diarrhea, cut back to a dose that does not produce it.

One caveat: After taking the powder form of vitamin C dissolved in water, rinse or brush your teeth, as the acidity can dissolve your tooth enamel.

If you want to double the power of your detox cocktail, add 600 milligrams (two 300 milligram capsules) of Lipoic Acid (Metabolic Maintenance). This is a superstar among antioxidants (Kagan). It is so powerful that it has reversed terminal liver disease. And I'm talking about people with less than a few days left to live due to accidental poison-mushroom ingestion, something medicine is powerless against (Teutsche, Becker, Berkson). In addition, lipoic acid is essential for gastric secretions (Harris), protects the pancreas from inflammatory damage (Burkart), and the liver from alcohol damage (Marshall).

There is no other nutrient in the detox cocktail that can do all that lipoic acid does. For example, it boosts the lifespan of vitamins C and E by recycling them and boosts glutathione synthesis, the main ingredient in Recancostat (Bast, Sen, Packer). It is a nutrient that you should have every day, in sickness or in health, and it adds a powerful punch to your detox cocktail.

Detox Enema

"Ugh! I don't do enemas, so I'll skip this section."

Just hold on a moment! I've heard every negative there is regarding enemas. But even more, I have heard folks chastise themselves for not doing the detox enema for years, only to discover that it provided instant relief. Then they wished they had done it sooner.

Granted, the word *enema* turns off many folks who say they could never even consider such a procedure. But I can attest to thousands of folks, myself included, for whom it has been a lifesaver. If you are sick in any way, and especially if you know you have ingested something that is flaring up in your gut, try it.

Whenever your body has an undesirable symptom, its ability to detoxify the daily onslaught has been surpassed. In contrast, when your detoxification system has all cylinders pumping, we can eat, drink, inhale, and be merry. The toxins and the total load of stressors to the body don't seem to faze us.

So, why not speed up the body's ability to detoxify by decreasing its workload? What's wrong with feeling your normal, energetic self, say after a night out on the town when you've eaten and drunk too much and are bloated and hungover as a result? That's what the detox enema does.

The last stage of detoxification occurs in your gut when chemicals from air, food, water, and uninvited germs march down to be excreted. Unfortunately, if they're not excreted soon enough, they can be reabsorbed, especially if the gut is leaky. This is one reason why folks with constipation feel so bad. As the stool bulks up within them, they reabsorb toxins and chemicals stored in the stool.

Such reabsorption will overburden an already compromised detox system, adding new symptoms to your usual ones. But if you can get rid of those toxins by enema, unloading your detox system as you do so, it will also allow you to clean up any other toxins that are making you sick. Now you can see why enemas can shorten the course of any illness, and in many cases folks feel better within an hour.

The procedure is simple. Get one enema bag (N.E.E.D.S.) and Folger's fully caffeinated coffee (red can). Pour four cups of filtered water into a pan, add two tablespoons of coffee, and bring to a boil for two minutes, then turn off the burner. Let it cool to baby-bottle temperature, gently warm. Pour liquid only (not the grounds) into the enema bag and hang it at waist level in the bathroom. Lie on the floor and insert the tube into the rectum. Unclamp the hose and let half (two cups) of the liquid flow into the rectum, then remove the tube. Rest and read something peaceful for ten minutes, then get up and expel the enema into the toilet. Repeat once. What could be simpler?

Liver and Gallbladder Flush

The liver and gallbladder flush does just that: flushes clean the liver, bile ducts, and gallbladder. Although this is a lengthy protocol, many folks do it once a year just to keep their gallbladders free of sludge and the tiny stones that can eventually grow into the larger, painful stones that require surgery.

The rationale here is to make the bloodstream very acidic for a few days so you can loosen the sludge and dissolve calcifications.

Anecdotal stories abound about how people have relieved themselves of sludge and stones and felt much better after doing the flush. In fact, hundreds of my patients who did the flush report excellent results. None have had problems with gallstones and none have had to have surgery. Nonetheless, it is possible that gallstones will require surgery, even on an emergency basis, for the unlucky few.

Calcium is one of the main buffers in the blood that neutralizes acid generated from processed foods, sodas, cigarettes, other chemical exposures, disease, allergic reactions, infection, bad thoughts, and much more. Yes, even bad or worrisome thoughts can trigger a release of body chemicals that need to be buffered or neutralized equal to that triggered by inhaling a bad chemical. This is one reason why peace of mind is so pivotal to your health.

When any of these triggers cause our cells to become too acidic, they become weak, lose important minerals, and start to malfunction. This is the beginning of chronic degenerative disease. So we need excellent stores of calcium, and bone makes a wonderful calcium bank. The problem is that many people have overdrawn on their calcium account, resulting in osteoporosis.

A bigger problem occurs with the way in which folks think they should be putting calcium back into the body. They take 500 to 1200 milligrams a day without properly balancing it with the other dozen minerals that are needed in order to hold the calcium in the bone. The result? Instead of shoring up the bones, the calcium calcifies or "hardens" the arteries of the brain and heart (arteriosclerosis), or makes kidney stones and gallstones.

Procedure for Liver Gallbladder Flush

Prepare a half ounce each of freshly squeezed lime juice and extra virgin olive oil. Drink this daily for one week. The next week, double the amount to an ounce of each and drink it daily. By the third week drink a mixture of one and a half ounces of each daily, until a tarry stool is passed. This should look darker than your normal stool, often black, and be less formed. This represents gallbladder sludge, and the flush is ended when this occurs.

For many folks, the liver and gallbladder flush has improved their liver's efficiency in detoxifying common substances. At the same time, it has relieved the gallbladder of accumulated sludge and smaller stones which could have gone on to form infection and larger, obstructing gallstones.

Parasympathetic Protocol

Your nervous system functions in two distinct ways. The *sympathetic nervous system* prepares you for fight or flight; it prepares you to defend yourself from an attacker, say, or to run like mad from a burning building. As most of the blood is shunted to your muscles and heart during such moments, the body must re-route blood from other areas that are not in so much need. As a result, the secretion of digestive juices slows to a halt, since blood is taken from the digestive tract.

The *parasympathetic nervous system,* on the other hand, energizes the glands, promotes healing and repair, and aids in digestion. So if you come home from a stressful day at the office, you must relax before you can reap the benefits of your parasympathetic nervous system.

If the TV is blaring with the latest action film interspersed with hard-sell commercials, for example, you may never get into the parasympathetic mode. Hence, when you go to bed a few hours later, the undigested bolus of food that never moved out of your stomach will begin to ferment and bubble up into the esophagus. Since you're lying prone when you sleep, it's all too easy for it to leak back up into the esophagus and cause severe heartburn and indigestion, even to the point of mimicking a heart attack.

Listen to soothing music, dim the lights, use unscented candles, have a relaxing conversation, give and receive a loving mini-massage, read a bit from your favorite book, take a warm bath, putter in the garden, play the piano or guitar, walk the dog, drink a cup of ginger tea, or watch a sunset: Do whatever you have to do to get into the parasympathetic mode *before* you begin to eat.

Never underestimate how intimately the gut is tied to the brain. In fact, the brain and emotions are as much a stimulant to the gut as is any food, bug, ulcer, or cancer. And the opposite is also true: The gut can stimulate other parts of the body (Mossiman, Iacono). Be that as it may, never forget that you have absolute control over how threatening you perceive anything to be and how extensively you are going to allow it to affect your GI tract functions.

Nutrition Protocol (Levels I, II, III)

Above and beyond needing L-glutamine to heal the leaky gut, enzymes to improve digestion, probiotics to restore the normal flora, herbals to correct intestinal dysbiosis and to soothe the gut, there are many nutrients we need to speed gut healing.

Folks with minimal symptoms need only minimal nutrients (level I), while folks with more serious gut problems require something more (level II). Folks with the most serious gut problems, like Crohn's disease or ulcerative colitis, may require resting the gut (level III) before following any protocols, in addition to taking every test listed in the next chapter. Often, those who are the sickest cannot tolerate anything by mouth. Meanwhile healing is delayed indefinitely until they get the missing nutrients they need. Because we are dealing with such a wide array of unknowns determined by each person's biochemistry the following example guidelines are quite general. Let's start then with a nutritional protocol for folks with minimal symptoms who need a nutritional boost.

Level I

Principle: A good multivitamin and mineral formulation, extra vitamin C to detoxify the gut (always cut back if it causes diarrhea or stomach irritation, and switch to a buffered vitamin C powder [Klaire, Tyler, ARG] if the pure ascorbic acid form feels like it burns), extra antioxidants, omega-3 essential fatty acids, and accessory factors to speed detoxification and healing.

Tyler Program
Multi-Plex-1 without iron, one to two capsules, twice a day
Buffered C Powder, a half to one teaspoon in a large eight-ounce glass of
    water, one to six times a day
Cyto-Redoxin, one to two capsules, twice a day
Eskimo-3, two capsules, twice a day
Detoxication Factors, one to two capsules, twice a day

Thorne Program
Basic Nutrients II, one to two capsules, twice a day
Pure Ascorbic Acid Powder or Capsules, a half to one teaspoon or one to
    three capsules with a large glass of water, one to four times a day
Plant Antioxidants, one to two capsules, twice a day
Super EPA, one to two capsules, twice a day
Phytisone, one capsule, twice a day

Carlson Program
Cardi-Rite, one to two capsules, twice a day
Mild-C Crystals, one-quarter to one teaspoon, once a day
ACES Gold, one to two capsules a day
Cod Liver Oil (Carlson): one teaspoon a day

Or you could choose an eclectic assortment of high-quality nutrients. In other words, you could chose the multiple from one supplier, the antioxidant from another, and the oils from yet another.

Level II

Folks who need to follow the level II protocol are a little more damaged and may need to add one or more nutrients to one of the above protocols.

Magnesium

Magnesium can help stop gut spasm. Use any one of the following:

Magnesium Chloride Solution 18% (Ecologic Formulas, ARG): A liquid, as bad as it tastes, is the fastest way to stop spasm due to magnesium deficiency, short of an intravenous infusion. The dose is one to two teaspoons twice a day in a large glass of water. For folks who hate the liquid form, other well-absorbed forms are listed below, although for emergencies or tough cases you cannot beat liquid.

K/Mg Citrate (Metabolic Maintenance), three to four capsules a day
Magnesium Citrate (Metabolic Maintenance), three capsules a day
Magnesium Citrate (Thorne), three capsules a day
Magnesium Aspartate (Thorne), three to six capsules a day
Magnesium Citrate + Potassium and Taurine (Jarrow), two capsules, twice a day

Chlorophyll

Chlorophyll to cleanse and detoxify the gut (use any one of the following):
Kyo-Green (Wakunaga), one to two heaping tablespoons in a large glass of good water, two to six times a day
Yaeyama Chlorella (Jarrow), four to ten capsules or two to three teaspoons, two to six times a day in juice or water

Methyl Sulfonyl Methane (MSM)

Methyl sulfonyl methane (MSM) provides sulfur for detoxification and for rebuilding tissues. When the gut is inflamed, we're talking about major rebuilding of an area the size of a tennis court. Some of my favorite sources are Jarrow and Longevity Science, powder or crystals, 500 milligrams, one to two, twice a day.

Arginine

L-arginine is an amino acid used by the body to repair tissues. L-Arginine (Jarrow), one to two of the 500 milligram capsules twice daily.

Thymus and Pituitary

One packet of Biopro-A Thymic (Longevity Science) dissolved and held under the tongue as long as possible three to five times a day speeds healing in many folks. Also, with its track record for nipping infections in the bud, it is useful to boost thymic immune function to aid in healing as well as defending the seriously inflamed gut from infection.

And for a pituitary extract, Pituitary Plus (Thorne), one to two capsules taken twice a day may further boost the immune system. When glandulars make no difference within a month, they are best dropped from the program to avoid turning off any normal function of the gland by feedback inhibition.

Phosphatidylcholine (PC)

I would be hard-pressed to decide which nutrients, phosphatidylcholine (PC) or fatty acids, are more important for repairing damaged membranes in the cell wall, detox area, and mitochondrial area. These areas represent the computer keyboard of the cell, the endoplasmic reticulum where detoxification takes place, and the mitochondrial organelles where energy is made respectively.

Repair of these specialized membranes requires two very important nutrients that are usually overlooked: the omega-3 fatty acids and pure PC. Deficiencies here are extremely common and must be corrected for complete healing of any organ to occur.

The omega-3 oils, EPA and DHA, are covered by your taking cod liver oil (Carlson) or Eskimo-3 (Tyler). And the best source of PC is Phos Chol Concentrate (American Lecithin)—one teaspoon contains 3000 milligrams of pure phosphatidylcholine. This form is so potent that studies at Massachusetts Institute of Technology have shown reversal of early Alzheimer's. All these oils are best refrigerated to extend shelf life.

It is important for you to include PC and omega-3 oils in your daily nutrient regimen if you are not healing. Lacking them may be what is holding you back, for they also help the body make more acetylcholinesterase, the very nerve-to-muscle transmitter that is stimulated by prescription drugs (Propulcid and Reglan) that have lots of nasty cardiac side effects. But PC cannot do anything harmful, for it is merely replenishing basic body building blocks and what is missing in the first place.

As always, when you incorporate nutritional medicine into your lifestyle, you not only avoid the bad side effects of drugs, but you get all sorts of good side effects thrown in. Things clear up that you never dreamed of getting rid of, because you didn't know what was missing in order to bring about a cure.

If you are very allergic to soy and cannot use Phos Chol Concentrate, use Soy-Free Phosphatides (Ecologic Formulas); take two to three capsules, twice a day.

Vitamin L?

Without sufficient vitamin L, the best treatments in the world can be a total flop. What is vitamin L? Love and laughter, which are even more important than any store-bought nutrient, for they make or break any program's success.

Level III

The level III regimen is for folks with the most serious gut diseases. For example, those with Crohn's disease, bloody colitis, and similar conditions take many prescription drugs to prevent them from having surgery. With so many food allergies to deal with, such folks also require injections to enable them to make blocking antibodies to the foods they're allergic to (described in *The E. I. Syndrome*), so they can eat them with fewer or no symptoms. At the same time, they must allow their gut to rest.

As a result, nourishment is obtained periodically either intravenously in the hospital or rectally at home. That gut cells heal rather fast, faster than most other cells in the body, is more than a stroke of luck. Thus, doing a daily retention enema for one week may provide such folks with a somewhat greater tolerance to the foods they're allergic to and help them moderate their drug use.

A retention enema can get needed nutrients into the body that otherwise would not be tolerated by the stomach or would be too expensive intravenously. As the name suggests, merely fill your enema bag (N.E.E.D.S. carries them), hang it on the bathroom door and lie down on the floor. Let one to two cups of the enema drip in at a time and hold it in for a half-hour or longer, if you are able. Better yet is to hold it for two to four hours, and best is not to expel it at all, so it all gets absorbed.

It works better if you use a water enema to cleanse the bowel first, evacuate, and then mix whatever retention enema you are using. Be sure to use good, clean (filtered, not tap) water. The loss of blood and mucus can cause dehydration quickly. One to four gallons could be needed. In one batch of water you could put your probiotics. Remember that you will only put in, at maximum, a quart or less each time. If you can elevate your hips on pillows six to twenty-four inches that will help the enema go higher and increase its chances of long retention. Until you get accustomed to how much you can retain and for how long, stay near the bathroom. It's not a time to go shopping.

Vitamin C powder, one to four teaspoons could go in another batch, or the Detoxification Factors, Permeability Factors, Enterogenic Factors, or any other probiotics. Obviously pull apart any capsules and empty their contents into the enema water. If the capsules cannot be pulled apart, prick them with a pin. Organic carrot juice and any green juice, like Kyo-Greens could go into the enema.

And if bowel-sparing, hydrolyzed, ready-to-absorb Sea Cure or Ultra-Clear cannot be tolerated by mouth, perhaps the rectal route will work. Use only solo products in an enema so it will be easier to evaluate your response. Also, make sure the product is well-diluted, using at least twice as much water as you would normally drink it with. A good rule of thumb is two cups of water for every dose of a nutrient, instilled for half an hour, getting rid of it only if you have to. The idea is to get as much absorbed via the rectal route as possible.

If it is the lower sigmoid area of the gut that is damaged, then by all means do not do any enemas, unless they are steroid (cortisone) enemas prescribed by your doctor. Instead, if that area is damaged, you will need to take the above by mouth. When the lower colon is very damaged by colitis, gastroenterologists prescribe cortisone enemas to tone down inflammation, which could lead to life-threatening bleeding. You don't want to take any chances of flaring up this damaged gut wall any more than it already is.

There is one exception: Once you have begun to heal the lower colon first with your prescription cortisone enemas, then use a butyric acid enema (Tyler), once or twice a day, as butyrate is extremely healing to the gut. In fact, it has caused colon cancer cells to redifferentiate, or revert to normal cells, in animal and human studies. If you must take a capsule form by mouth, use Cal-Mag Butyrate (Ecologic Formulas), taking one to six after meals.

A third option that can be included with any of the above or alone would be BottomsUp (ARG/Nutricology/Purity Products). It contains 15 grams of vitamin C, 30 multi-equivalents of magnesium chloride, 2 milliliters of trace minerals, 2 grams of taurine, 600 milligrams of glutathione, and 2 milliliters of B complex.

The protocol for administration is to clean the bowel first with a water enema. Then, using a 500 millileter Pyrex measuring cup, pour in 100 milliliters of the solution. Add 400 milliliters of clean water and one-eighth to one-quarter teaspoon of sea salt. Instill via enema bag into the rectum. In contrast to the detox enema, hang the bag as high as you can get it (on a coat hanger over the top of the door or on the shower head will do).

Bending the knees while lying on your back, raise your hips a foot or more off the floor so that you can get the enema solution as high in the colon as possible. Once it is in, relax and massage your belly for a few moments. Then (with enema tip removed) go about your business and try to retain the solution in the rectum as long as possible, preferably for more than two hours. Doing this twice daily, if tolerated, can boost healing of the gut immeasurably.

If you do a retention enema of glutamine (use two teaspoons of L-glutamine powder in two cups of good, filtered water), be sure to do it two hours away from any other enemas, as acidity inactivates it. It has been found to be incredibly safe (Hornsby-Lewis, Ziegler).

The Total Load

A damaged gut, or any other organ/system of the body, is never caused by a deficiency of some drug. Healing involves a three-stage process: (1) identify the triggers, like invading organisms, nutrient deficiencies, or hidden allergies; (2) unload the detoxification system so that healing or rebuilding can be a priority; then (3) protect the system so that you never get into trouble again.

Unloading the detox system can be as simple as washing a cut before you put a bandage on it. It includes anything you do that reduces the amount of work the body has to do in order to bring about healing.

Imagine two men who were badly damaged in an auto accident, lying side by side in a hospital room. Both receive identical care. The only difference is that one eats burgers and fries, and drinks Cokes all day, while the other has whole, nutritious, live foods—plenty of raw fruits and vegetables each day plus whole grain and bean dishes. He also snacks on nuts and seeds. Which one would you bet your last dollar on for healing faster?

Many studies show that you can cut the healing time in half (and the number of hospital days in half) with the addition of a multiple-vitamin supplement each day, which costs mere pennies a day. This is one more way of reducing the total amount of work the system has to do so it has enough energy with which to heal.

So avoid narrowly focusing on the gut when you are healing. Be sure to assess your total load of factors in your life. Do you get enough sleep? A nap during tough healing times can really boost your efforts. And you can tell you needed it when it becomes a dead sleep, something you would normally never be capable of in the middle of the day.

Do you get enough sunshine, fresh air, exercise and/or yoga stretches? Do you drink enough water? Do you surround yourself with loving friends, giving back more nurturing than you get? And do you connect with God? Scores of studies (in *Depression Cured At Last!*) show that folks with a sound spirituality heal faster and with fewer complications than others.

Environmental Controls

By now you know that if the gut isn't healthy, you haven't much hope of completely healing any other parts of your body. How can you prevent recurrent infections, for instance, when your body is too busy detoxifying toxins in the gut? How can you prevent an early heart attack or chemical mutation of your genetics that may allow a cancer to grow and spread when you cannot fully absorb the nutrients you need? This list could go on but I'm sure you see my point.

On the other hand, if you do have an ailing gut but no other symptoms, don't be fooled into thinking everything else is well. You will succumb to nutrient deficiencies from your ailing gut sooner than you think. Add to this the side effects from the drugs you'll take in response to your gut problems, the progression of the undiagnosed cause, or the many symptoms stemming from a Candida outbreak or a leaky gut, just to name two, and the danger grows.

The gut lining contains half of the body's capacity to detoxify and over half of the body's immune system. If anything goes wrong here, your vulnerability to disease including cancer, will certainly increase. My perspective on this is very clear: A healthy gut is key to cancer prevention and all successful cancer treatment.

Even the pancreas, so important to the GI system, is vital for protection from and healing of cancer. Why? It has to do with how the immune system and cancer cells interact. As I've mentioned before, the immune system does not "see" cancer cells, which possess a mucus protein coat over their antigenic recognition sites.

That's where pancreatic enzymes come in: They can dissolve the mucus coat, enabling the immune system to locate and attack cancer cells. Why then do we have so much more cancer than ever before in the history of mankind? Enter dwindling pancreatic function compromised by diets high in sweets, processed foods, fat, poor intestinal function, late meals, stress, intestinal medications, the wrong intestinal flora, pesticides, and environmental chemicals.

Yes, the proper treatment for every gut symptom, regardless of how seemingly innocent it may appear, has far-reaching effects on total health and longevity. But because an important detoxification system lines the gut, the reverse is also true. If the detox system has too much work to do generally, you will retard the healing of the gut in response.

So, take care that your total load does not force your detox system into overload. Even the little things can help here because they all add up. For instance, make sure that you live in the cleanest environment—which includes the air you breathe, the food you eat, and the water you drink—that you can.

1. Install a water filter on the sink for cleaner drinking water (such as from the American Health Foundation). The catalogs in the Resource Guide provide many fine sources.
2. Use an air purifier for the bedroom, where you spend a third of your life. You can also get them in a variety of sizes for your car and office (E. L. Foust Co., 1-800-225-9549, and many more sources in Chapter 8).

3. Use all-cotton bedding (KB Cotton Pillows, Janice's).
4. Eat fewer processed foods containing additives, dyes, and preservatives.
5. Refer to many more tips in my previous books *The E.I. Syndrome, Tired Or Toxic?, Wellness Against All Odds*, and *Depression Cured At Last!*

And remember: (1) failure to be aware of and to address the total load of stressors that your body has to deal with is a major reason why some folks will never get better; (2) an overloaded detox system will back up and delay or even prevent healing anywhere in the body.

CHAPTER 7

Sorting Through the Mountain
of Causes

By using the protocols described in preceding chapters most folks will be able to get themselves well. If, on the other hand, you have a relentless gut that just won't quit aggravating you, you will need diagnostic tests to pin down why.

I'll start where most of gastroenterology leaves off: after X rays of the gut accompanied by chalky-tasting solutions to drink or enemas plus scopes that peek into each end of the gut. Beyond those tests, there seems little more that traditional medicine can do. When ulcers, colitis, or cancers have not shown up, doctors usually fall back on the catch-all diagnosis: irritable bowel syndrome (IBS). A fallback diagnosis, however, is worthless if you are counting on finding a cause and cure. It merely returns you to a lifetime of drugs, whose side effects you learned about in Chapter 1.

Caveat: The Less Likely Causes

There are a multitude of other causes for chest and abdominal symptoms that can mimic indigestion from hepatitis and gastric cancer to heart or lung disease. And the list is far from complete without mention of pancreatic cancer; Zollinger-Ellison syndrome; cystic fibrosis; abdominal aneurysm; ectopic pregnancy; problems with the uterus, ovaries, prostate, kidney, liver, or back bones; leukemia or lymphoma; carcinoid syndrome; angioedema; sickle cell abdominal crisis; acute intermittent porphyria; hemochromatosis from too much beer or wine; motility defect from diabetes; or constipation from hypothyroidism, as examples.

Nausea that confounds the most astute diagnostician can be the only symptom of a brain tumor. I will assume you have ruled these out. The lucky part for you is that the vast majority of causes fall into the realm that you have learned about here and that you have direct control over. Don't be frightened by this list, but let it remind you that you are not a physician and there is a great deal more to be learned than could ever fit in one book. When you doubt the diagnosis that your doctor has given you, never hesitate to consult a specialist for a second opinion. If you are still getting sicker and finding no relief at this point, then your gut may be the cause. In the meantime, the odds are in your favor of your having plain old irritable bowel or heartburn caused by what I have described for you here.

General Guidelines

There is no absolute order of tests. The tests for individual gut conditions are outlined in the previous chapter. If you think you have Candida overgrowth because you have had many antibiotics and you have all the symptoms described in Chapter 3, then get the 7-Day Candida Culture ordered. If the test is positive but you are no better after you treat the Candida, then check to see if it is still there or do a comprehensive digestive stool analysis (CDSA) to find out what other bugs are present. Remember that is how you peel back the layers of the onion to find all the causes. If you are still no better but you realize you could have something harmful growing in your gut, then do the Purged Parasites test.

Since all gut conditions can mimic one another, the best guide is to keep working through the tests until you find the causes. When you have ruled out any abnormal organisms through CDSA, 7-Day Candida Culture, and Purged Parasites, persistent symptoms would dictate that you do a leaky gut test for intestinal hyperpermeability. But bear in mind that most folks will not need to do so many tests.

So use the guide in the previous chapter to determine what tests you need or follow the treatment protocols and methods for symptomatic relief that I have provided. Recall that some tests are available through only one lab in the country while other tests are offered by a variety of labs. Use the lab that is best for you. They are all of excellent quality or I would not have referred you to them. Coincidentially, be sure to check your medical insurance options to help you decide which labs best meet your health and financial needs.

Pinning Down the Causes

Now for the practical part of what tests to have, when and why, as well as where to get them. First, you must have a prescription from your doctor with the name of the test on it and your diagnosis. (Usually IBS, 564.1, is sufficient, which merely means irritable bowel syndrome.)

Next, select a lab from the Resource Guide and call the 800 number for the lab that does the test. Request that they send you the kit for the test on your prescription. When you receive it, read all directions carefully. For the tests that can be done at home, requiring urine or stool, read the instructions twice, then map out your course of action by making notes on the times you are to do certain things. If the test calls for blood or samples that you cannot get at home, go to any lab, hospital, or blood-drawing station and have your blood drawn, being sure that they have followed the directions supplied with the kit. I cannot overemphasize that you must be the captain of the ship, for yours may be the first kit like this that your lab has ever seen. Again, read all directions carefully *before* you show up at the lab. Do not expect them to be proficient in these tests or to take the time to carefully read all the directions. For over a decade I have seen lab technicians make every error conceivable, mainly because they did not want to take the time to read the directions enclosed in the kits.

Once the appropriate specimens are labeled in their containers, check whatever else has to be done (including payment) and return it all, including your prescription, in the prepaid mailer. If the lab does not receive payment and a prescription, the tests will not be performed.

Within a few weeks the physician who wrote the prescription will receive the results. If you want another physician to consult on the results as well, you can request a copy from the ordering physician and send it on.

So what tests are available to every doctor that your physician has not ordered? The following tests for folks with gut problems are offered by **Great Smokies Diagnostic Laboratory:**

Comprehensive Digestive and Stool Analysis (CDSA)

CDSA uncovers what bad bugs, including Candida, are growing in the gut. It also tells about other functions, such as digestion and absorption. I recall a time when, if I took so much as a sip of water, my stomach felt like a load of rocks had been dumped into it. CDSA showed that I had picked up Klebsiella, a bacteria that commonly causes irritable bowel symptoms. Klebsiella can be picked up in food from restaurants, packaged foods, or foods that have spoiled. Within three days of treatment, the months of mysterious symptoms that had plagued me disappeared for good.

CDSA is an easy test to do. Once you get the prescription and the kit, you need only follow the directions at home, putting your stool in the containers included in the kit.

The results indicate if you have defective digestion or absorption, as well as what unwanted bacteria and fungi are growing in your gut. Let's take a closer look at some common examples.

Interpreting the Results of the CDSA

One measurement determines if you have above-normal amounts of undigested food fiber. If you note there is above-normal vegetable or meat fibers or triglycerides, this can mean you have poor pancreatic function, low stomach acid, poor chewing, or bile salt deficiency.

If the level of the digestive enzyme chymotrypsin is low, this also suggests a bad diet, or low pancreatic or gastric secretions. For more information on chymotrypsin-containing digestive enzymes, refer to the enzyme protocol section in the preceding chapter.

Certainly, low thyroid (i.e., hypothyroidism, a cause of sluggish bowel) or mineral and vitamin deficiencies, or even an intestinal blockage can also produce low chymotrypsin levels. To determine cause here, ask your clinician to sort through all of your history and physical findings and then combine what he or she has learned from all your tests, and decide on the most likely alternative. For practical purposes, I'll deal with the most likely alternatives here.

A high chymotrypsin level can indicate the presence of abnormal bugs in the gut, gluten intolerance (wheat, oats, rye, and barley antigens), food allergies, and pancreatic malfunction. For more information on a gluten-free diet and food allergy diagnostic diet, refer to Chapter 2. For more information on how to treat abnormal bugs, refer to Chapter 3. For more information on how to use digestive enzymes, refer to Chapter 6. **Remember:** even high levels of pancreatic chymotrypsin can be triggered by abnormal bugs, which can be controlled by the ingestion of various herbs, as well as by digestive enzymes. As a result, while with high levels you should not need an enzyme you still must always try to keep the underlying cause in sight.

If the acid/base balance, or pH, is high, it can indicate an insufficient amount of good bugs, low stomach acid, ammonia production from a high-meat diet, or slow bowel transit time (usually from inadequate fiber intake). For more information on how probiotics can replenish the good bugs, refer to Chapter 4. You can also refer to Chapter 6 to determine how protiotics can replenish stomach acid by digestives containing betaine HCl.

If the pH is low, meaning on the acidic side, again consider bacterial

Table 14. Quick Guide to Finding the protocols in Previous Chapters

Protocol	Chapter
Diagnostic diet for hidden food allergies	2
Candida	3
Paragard	3
H. pyloris	4
Probiotic	4
Intestinal dysbiosis (unwanted gut bugs)	4
DGL (Rhizinate)	4
Leaky gut syndrome	5
Pure Body Program	5
Vitamin C flush	5
Magnesium flush	5
Fiber cleansing protocol	6
Digestive enzymes	6
Detox cocktail	6
Detox enema	6
Gallbladder flush	6
Parasympathetic protocol	6
Nutrition protocol	6
Total load	6
Environmental controls	6

overgrowth, poor pancreatic function, or rapid bowel transit time as culprits. If you cannot identify the bugs, refer to the Paragard trial as described in Chapter 3 for a possible solution. The pancreatic enzyme trial can be of aid here as well in solving a lack of pancreatic enzymes. Fast transit time of stool through the gut has many potential causes, from food allergy to bad bugs.

Let's turn now from digestive function, to digestive absorption. You can have the greatest set of chompers and terrific digestive enzymes, but if the gut is inflamed from food allergies, Candida overgrowth, or gluten enteropathy (celiac disease), you won't absorb what you have gone to the trouble to digest. For example, a CDSA that shows cholesterol, or the long-chain fatty acids, to be elevated can point to malabsorption from a variety of causes, from bad bugs or nutrient deficiencies to food allergy or medication damage (as from nonsteroidal anti-inflammatory drugs [NSAIDs] like Motrin, Aleve, Advil) that causes leaky gut.

Elevated levels of short-chain fatty acids of n-butyrate can also signify any of these, as well as rapid transit time or pancreatic insufficiency; depressed levels are commonly caused by bad bugs (usually resulting from overgrowth after antibiotics), insufficient fiber or water, or slow transit time. Since butyrates are one of the preferred sources of energy for repairing gut cells, they're used as an indicator of gut content health, with emphasis on absorption. Probiotics, Paragard protocol, and digestive enzymes may be the simple solutions, singularly or together.

If levels of the enzyme beta glucuronidase are elevated, it could mean inflammation, colon cancer, abnormal nutrient levels and bugs, or a high-meat diet. High levels can secondarily cause an increased risk for breast cancer for women on estrogens. Low levels usually indicate abnormal bugs, usually from antibiotics. This enzyme has far too many functions in the gut to explain, but suffice it to say that you definitely do not want it to be high, as it revs up the absorption of gut carcinogens (chemicals that can cause cancer).

Secretory immunoglobulin A (sIgA) is a special antibody produced in the saliva and gut. It is the first line of defense against bad bugs in the gut. If sIgA levels are too low, it is often because the immune system has become overwhelmed by too many bad bugs, nutrient deficiencies, or both. High levels of sIgA indicate a need to fight off extra amounts of infection, although they also signify that you are rallying to the cause. High sIga levels could also be in response to a bacterial toxin, for the gut is the last place for toxins to concentrate in during their passage out of the body. Researchers have also shown that a particularly low sIgA level can be a sign of, and a result of, food allergy as the inflammation compromises sIgA secretion (Brandtzeg).

Now the fun part of the CDSA test: the bacteria or bugs. One of the most common bacteria seen is Klebsiella—which can cause arthritis, irritable bowel symptom, and leaky gut—followed by Citrobacter, Pseudomonas, Proteus, Salmonella, Bacillus, and *Staphylococcus aureus*. They can mimic any gut symptom as well as present with a baffling array of other body symptoms, which can only be appreciated because they leave when the bug is treated.

Clostridia, a particularly nasty bacteria will usually overgrow as a result of taking antibiotics. Once Clostridia gets a foothold, it can cause severe diarrhea and even colitis.

Whenever there is overgrowth of specific bacteria, it indicates several things: (1) probable antibiotic use which has upset the flora; (2) poor body defenses to fight it off, including digestive and nutrient deficiencies; (3) poor diet; or (4) undetected food allergies. However, worse is the fact that (5) for every bug that is found in abnormally high numbers, there may be others that did not show up this time, as we peel back layers of the onion to reveal what is lurking beneath.

An assay like this can only reveal the predominating bugs. Since there are over 500 varieties of bugs in the gut, it is beyond the scope of any lab to give a count on them all. As a result, only the most prevalent bugs are picked up first. After the leader of the pack has been killed, however, it is not at all uncommon to discover another nasty bug on a second test that did not show up before.

Folks will often ask in alarm where they could have gotten such bugs. Recall that volumes of studies show that city water across the United States is frequently contaminated, as are foods, especially meats, fowl, and fish. In addition, eating out as much as we Americans do adds even more risk factors, not to mention our increased travel to foreign lands and the importation of foreign foods into our local supermarkets. Top this off with our hefty ritual of taking antibiotics for every sneeze and wheeze, and you will be left asking yourself how we do as well as we do.

Knowing how many and what types of the good bacteria are present is also important. This test, the mycology assay, tells if there are sufficient good bacteria present or if you should do the probiotic protocol to attain sufficiency. Aim for 4+ *lactobacillus* and 4+ *bifidus*. You want the maximum amount of good bugs to boost the immune system of the gut lining. (See Chapter 4.)

If abnormal amounts of yeasts or fungi, like Candida, are found on the mycology assay then it's probably an overgrowth of *Candida albicans*. Folks may want to see if improper treatment of their presumed Candida has resulted in an overgrowth of the Nystatin-resistant form, *Candida tropicalis*. Of course, we often see that it is really *Rhodotorula* or another fungus, *Geotrichum,* that is creating all the havoc. *Rhodotorula* and *Geotrichum* are treated the same as Candida and like Candida, can be picked up on CDSA, 7-Day Candida Culture, or Purged Parasites test.

So there you have the highlights of one bowel test that the majority of doctors do not even know about, much less order, and few, if any, hospitals perform. Stick to your guns and get what I consider to be one of the most valuable gut tests going. No other test provides so much front-line information about the function of your gut as the CDSA.

Leaky Gut Test

After reading Chapter 5, you'll want to know if you have leaky gut syndrome (LGS). But if your doctor won't order the appropriate test, treating it yourself is safe and can give you an answer, especially if it requires only the most elementary level of regimens. For example, if you suspect you have leaky gut and put yourself on L-glutamine powder (as described in Chapter 5) for a month and find your gut symptoms disappearing, you probably had leaky gut and successfully treated it. If that does not begin to bring relief, then your reading should give you a rough idea of whether or not you could be harboring Candida or other bugs, in which case you owe it to yourself to do the Candida or Paragard protocol for a month.

The test for leaky gut, or intestinal permeability, requires an extra step. You must get two prescriptions: (1) one for the leaky gut test and (2) one that says "intestinal permeability test solutions, disp. 100 cc, sig. As dir." With both prescriptions in your possession, turn to the one that says "leaky gut test," call the lab, and get the kit. Follow the directions carefully, especially those that explain when to drink the solution and how to collect your urine specimen and return it with your prescription. The test involves two urine tests that you will collect at home. Take the first urine sample before you drink the test solution, and then take the second urine sample after drinking the test solution.

To do the test you need a lactulose-mannitol solution to drink. It is this solution that combines two sugars, lactulose and mannitol, which, as they appear in your urine, determine how leaky or malabsorptive your gut is. The pharmacies that mail the solution are also listed in the Resource Guide. In some states, the solution comes from the lab, so ask the lab to provide it along with your kit when you place the order.

Yes, the test solution contains two sugars, and thousands of recovering Candida victims have been afraid to take it because of their fear of triggering Candida again. Not to fear though: One dose is not sufficient to cause a recurrence, unless you are close to having a recurrence anyway. In that case, the test is all the more necessary, especially in regard to how vulnerable you are to a multitude of nasty Candida-related symptoms, in addition to how leaky is your gut. If you are that near the edge that one drink will set you back, chances are even greater that your gut wall has been damaged from untreated Candida or other intestinal dysbioses.

Interpreting Results of the Leaky Gut Test

As with all tests, the results come with an interpretation, which is mailed to the doctor who prescribed them. If there is an increased amount of either sugar in the urine, a leakiness is indicated. The increase is easily seen on the report as a numerical value as well as in graph form. If there is an insufficient amount of either sugar, there is some level of malabsorption. The gut status is more obvious when both parameters are either too high (leaky) or too low (malabsorption). If only one value is abnormal and the other is not, then this merits treatment. There are many ways nutrients get absorbed across the gut wall. This test only looks at two of them. **Remember:** much guesswork is clarified when you find the underlying cause. Next, of course, you would want to do the CDSA to determine what infectious organisms (intestinal dysbiosis) might have triggered leakiness, or what digestive deficiencies might be contributing to the cause.

The most common cause of malabsorption is gluten enteropathy (celiac disease), a serious disease that usually requires immediate treatment to offset the weight loss that occurs each day. Carefully follow the directions for the wheat-, rye-, oats-, and barley-free diet in Chapter 2. The most commonly encountered causes for leakiness include food allergy, NSAIDs arthritis and pain medications, Crohn's disease (ulcerative colitis), alcoholism, abnormal bugs or deficiencies of digestive secretions.

7-Day Candida Culture or Candida Intensive Culture

For folks who already know they have or had Candida and merely need to follow up on that one organism the 7-Day Candida Culture is for them. Because this test costs only a fraction of the cost of the complete CDSA, it also saves money.

Merely have your physician write a prescription for it and call the lab for the kit. It is another stool test that you can do at home and return with the prescription to the lab. As the lab will return results to your physician, request that he or she provide you with a copy of the test and any help in interpreting it.

Interpreting the 7-Day Candida Culture

Having been blessed with the opportunity to work with thousands of Candida sufferers, I believe that no amount of reported Candida is tolerable. Physicians will argue that certainly we all have many types of fungi that are in happy balance with the hundreds of other organisms in the gut. This is correct. But we are the first generation of humans to have consumed so many antibiotics, not only ourselves, but via the animals we eat, which are raised on antibiotics routinely. With more than 500 organisms in the gut to rot or digest our food, there are many beneficial ones, but it is absurd to think that the presence of Candida, a cause of an alarming array of symptoms, is "normal and harmless." The proof of the pudding is that when I have treated patients with a reported 1+ Candida, a multitude of symptoms nearly always improved.

Again, know that the medical determination of "normal and harmless" for a reported 1+ Candida is wrong. Just because Candida is so prevalent does not in any way mean that it is normal.

Bottom line: I strongly recommend that you do not settle for anything less than absolutely no yeast forms found on the 7-Day Candida Culture, the CDSA, or the Purged Parasites test. Even if the phrase "rare yeast on KOH" appears on any report, with no specification regarding the type, I treat it. The gut is not meant to be a fungus field! With all the good bugs that should be present in a normal gut, there is no reason why a shallow look into the pond of the gut should show Candida as a predominating bug. Candida levels should never be high enough to be seen as one of the top ten bugs, nor should Candida be strong enough to grow through all the hundreds of other much more desirable and beneficial bugs.

The lab reports bugs in an arbitrary 1+, 2+, 3+, or 4+ system. So if you have 4+ Candida, you are in deep trouble, for that is as high as the lab can report. Who knows if you have the highest numbers ever seen by the lab. But as I warn, do not be hoodwinked by "low levels" of 1+ or "rare yeast" reports, either.

Sometimes the report says "no Candida found" but in the bottom right-hand edge of the report it will also say "rare yeast forms found." To me, this must be interpreted to mean that some type of fungus is present in high amounts and you should try to get rid of it. Once more, my conviction on this issue does not come lightly, but from treating hundreds of patients with reported "low" or "insignificant" levels of yeast, and observing the long-standing gut symptoms, as well as other conditions, dramatically disappear during treatment. For the protocol, refer to Chapter 3.

Comprehensive Parasitology or Purged Parasites

This test looks for parasites that usually do not show up on a CDSA, like giardia, amoeba, strongyloides, blastocystis, cryptosporidium, and others. Many such parasites are more prevalent contaminants of drinking water and foods in the United States. Thirty years ago when I was in medical school, we rarely thought of such parasites, unless someone had been out of the country. Now you need not go anywhere to get some of the most exotic parasites. The Comprehensive Parasitology test, or Purged Parasites test, is particularly useful when you know something is infected, but you cannot find the cause on CDSA.

As an added bonus, sometimes I will pick up Candida or other yeasts on this test, even though they were not found on the CDSA. That is because the word *purged* refers to a laxative that you took first, allowing the stool sample to come from higher up in the colon and even the small intestine— at times the exclusive residence of some unwanted bugs.

Have your physician write a prescription for the test. Call the lab for the kit, carefully follow the directions for putting stool in the kit, and return it to the lab in the mailer.

Folks are often surprised that they could have gotten some of these strange-sounding organisms, having no idea how contaminated our world has become. Cryptosporidium has become the most harmful contaminant found in treated city drinking water in the United States. And in the immunocompromised, like the elderly, or those fighting cancer and other diseases requiring nasty drugs (like steroids and chemotherapy) that intentionally weaken the immune system, cryptosporidium carries as high as a 68 percent mortality rate (Rose). That means that in every hundred folks who are immunocompromised and who drink water contaminated with cryptosporidium, sixty-eight will die. Think about it!

Interpreting the Purged Parasites Test

Parasites that show up on the Purged Parasites test are difficult to get rid of and may require prescription medications. Many safer herbal remedies, however, do exist, and should you try them first you may find that they work for you as well. Your best choice here is artemisia (Artecin), at full strength. (See Chapters 3, 5, 6, and the Resource Guide.) And again, when you see yeasts of any sort on this test, treat them!

Quantitative *H. pylori* Antibodies

This simple blood test shows if you have ever been infected with *Helicobacter pylori,* the bacterium that can cause gastritis or ulcers, turn off stomach acid secretion by causing the lining to deteriorate (atrophic gastritis), or cause stomach cancer.

Again, folks wonder *where* they could have picked up *H. pylori*, but it is more appropriate to wonder how we can *avoid* picking it up. Look at how frequently we pick up a newspaper or magazine to find an article about some new contaminant in beef, sprouts, chicken, municipal water supplies, or processed foods. For example, one government committee reported that campylobacter (**remember:** this is the other name for *H. pylori,* which you learned about in Chapter 4) was the leading bacterial pathogen in Minnesota, especially in the months of June through August, and that it was becoming more resistant to antibiotics. *H. pylori* is clearly becoming more prevalent than before even though it was already the leading cause of foodborne illness (Clapp).

Of course, you know by now one of the reasons why infection is becoming more prevalent. As soon as folks feel any gastric distress, all too many will reach for Mylanta or other antacids that sop up the natural stomach antibiotic, hydrochloric acid (HCl). And when this fails, they go to stronger medications like Tagamet or Zantac to more efficiently turn off acid production. This effectively adds fertilizer to the bug by wiping out our natural bug destroyer.

Interpretating the **H. pylori** *Test*

If the level of *H. pylori* is positive (elevated above normal) or if it is negative (normal) but you have a strong suspicion that you have infection, repeat the test in three to eight weeks. If the second level is the same, it most likely reflects an old disease, not a current infection. If the second level is lower, this means you are effectively getting rid of the bug. For when there is less of the bug present, your body responds by making fewer antibodies, hence the level, or titer, of anti-*H. pylori* antibodies is reduced. There is one exception here though: if you're getting lower levels because your body is just too weak to mount a defense any longer. This is a real danger sign of a failing immune system and requires immediate medical intervention. In this case you would be extremely ill, and your doctor should test your ability to mount an antibody response by measuring your antibody levels and your response to delayed and immediate skin test results. (He or she may prefer to refer you to an immunologist or allergist for these assays. As well, the intervention could be quite serious, for example, requiring a series of intravenous gamma globulin injections. If you are this sick, you have many other problems that have probably taken priority over the gut, like a cancer. In fact, it could be chemotherapy that has wiped out your ability to mount an antibody response.)

If the result of the second test is higher, it indicates that your body is making even more antibodies to the bug than before, in which case you most likely have an active infection that requires treatment. This is when you and your physician decide if you want to evaluate your response to one of the safer treatments in Chapter 4 or go straight to the triple antibiotics currently used in conventional drug-driven medicine. Whichever you decide, I would urge you to monitor blood levels to be sure they are getting lower every month or two, verifying that your treatment is succeeding. Whatever the results, be sure to check the level again in a year to be sure the infection has not recurred—recurrence is very common (and so is resultant gastric cancer).

Nutrient Deficiencies Keep Folks from Healing

You have just learned about the important gut studies not routinely done in medicine. Folks who resist healing despite the regimens and protocols they adopt, however, still need to find out why. Undiagnosed mineral, vitamin, and fatty-acid deficiencies lead the pack. You might find it as difficult as I did two decades ago to believe that healthy-looking folks living in the land of plenty could be deficient in this regard. Yet, it is rare to find anyone these days who does not have at least one or more deficiencies. And even if they feel fine now, they are an accident waiting to happen.

For example, government studies show that the average American gets only 40 percent of his or her daily requirement of magnesium. Other studies show that over 54 percent of patients in the hospital have a magnesium deficiency (Whang). Worse yet, the same study showed that 90 percent of doctors caring for these hospitalized folks did not even look for a magnesium deficiency, even in those who were dying of it. Was this *Journal of the American Medical Association* article mentioned on CNN? No! It was all but ignored, as doctors do not routinely test for magnesium status in severely ill patients. In the rare instance when a test is done, doctors usually do the least sensitive test of magnesium status available, the serum magnesium (for folks who want a lot more detail about this very important issue, complete with all the scientific references, see my book *Depression Cured At Last!*)

Another study showed that 39 percent of the populace got less than 70 percent of the daily requirement for magnesium (Marier). And is it any wonder, when studies prove that you can lose over 79 percent of the magnesium in going from whole wheat to white bleached flour? (Schroeder). In fact, it is our reliance on flour products, alcohol, and processed foods, all low in magnesium, that contributes to our epidemic of potentially fatal magnesium deficiency.

Add to this the fact that sugar, phosphates (chemicals common in processed foods, especially in soft drinks), alcohol, stress, and high-fat diets further lower magnesium levels (Seelig), and you see why authorities think at least 80 percent of the populace is magnesium deficient. Recall that magnesium deficiency can provoke interminable gut spasms (spastic colon), constipation, resistant cardiac arrhythmia, or sudden cardiac death. Because magnesium is pivotal to over 300 enzymes in the body, magnesium deficiencies can mimic nearly any symptom you can think of.

Mineral and Toxic Metal Analysis

The mineral and toxic metal analysis, properly called Elemental Analysis in Packed Erythrocytes or RBC Minerals, examines the levels of eight minerals and seven toxic heavy metals. The erythrocyte is the red blood cell (rbc) that floats in our serum to carry oxygen to our cells. The minerals this test analyzes from inside the red blood cell include magnesium, manganese, molybdenum, potassium, selenium, vanadium, and zinc. These minerals are important, as vanadium and zinc deficiencies, for example, can decrease pancreatic function. The heavy metals, or toxic elements, analyzed include cadmium, antimony, mercury, lead, silver, thallium, and tin. These heavy metals can slowly accumulate in the body over years of exposure to auto exhaust, dental fillings and porcelain crowns, canned foods, processed foods, pesticides, paints, plastics, and more.

Heavy metals can mimic any symptom you can think of from chronic fatigue to fibromyalgia, or prompt many diagnosed conditions like chronic Candida overgrowth or cancer resistant to treatment. Heavy metals accumulate inside cells, and more specifically inside the enzymes of cells where they substitute for minerals that belong in the enzymes. Because this seriously damages enzyme function, any type of malfunction is possible here, including any gut symptoms. The diagnosis starts with finding elevated heavy metals in the mineral test. Although treatment for heavy metal toxicity requires extensive discussion (as in *Wellness Against All Odds*), eating a healthier diet and correcting nutrient deficiencies for starters can bring many folks back to better health while deciding how to treat their heavy metal problem.

Ask your doctor for an RBC Minerals prescription, then call the lab for the test kit yourself. Take the kit to any local laboratory so they can draw the blood according to the instructions in the kit and then send it back to the lab for analysis. You doctor will get the written report, which you can request a copy of and help in interpreting.

Another analysis can be done from plasma instead of packed red blood cells. This assay also includes the toxic element aluminum. Recall how aluminium accumulates after years of eating out, years of taking antacids like Maalox or Mylanta, or the aluminum in salt and other foods to help them pour easier in spite of moisture. To determine your levels of aluminium toxicity, just order RBC Minerals from plasma.

You may wonder why mineral assays are available for inside the red blood cell and for minerals floating freely in the plasma or blood itself. The reason is simple: The body compartmentalizes its minerals. For example, some minerals go inside bone, some go inside certain types of cells, some go inside enzymes, and some go inside the cell membrane. When a deficiency crops up, the body robs Peter to pay Paul. If, for example, you are deficient in zinc, you could have a pancreatic digestive enzyme deficiency as well as a deficiency of carbonic anhydrase, the enzyme needed for making gastric HCl for digestion. With one deficiency of zinc, you have knocked out two important digestive enzymes.

With so little zinc to go around, the body may decide it needs to prioritize: It may keep zinc inside the liver cell for another enzyme, like alkaline phosphatase; or it may keep most of the zinc floating freely in the blood-stream so that it can be shuttled more quickly to whichever area most urgently needs it. Now you can appreciate how a test of serum zinc can look normal, while the rbc zinc test shows zinc as severely deficient. For this reason, the more areas you can measure minerals in, the better. But if you are strapped and can afford only one mineral assay, make sure it is for inside the cells, not the serum or plasma, for the body keeps most of its deficient minerals scouting through the serum on the lookout for areas that need to be rescued the most. It is by looking at the minerals inside the cells that you can see how severely deficient in minerals you really are.

Comprehensive Vitamin Profile

The comprehensive vitamin profile measures seventeen vitamins: beta-carotene, biopterin, biotin, carnitine, free choline, total choline, folic acid, inositol, niacin, pantothenic acid, riboflavin, thiamin, vitamin C, vitamin B_{12}, vitamin B_6, and vitamin E. As with the other tests, all you need is a prescription, then call the lab, get the kit, take it to the nearest blood-drawing station, and you're done.

Be careful if you are found to be deficient in a vitamin but taking it makes no difference. You probably are deficient in a particular enzyme that converts that vitamin to an active form, in which case you definitely would benefit from the expertise of a doctor proficient in nutritional chemistry. (Sources provided in the Resource Guide.)

Essential and Metabolic Fatty Acids Analysis

If you think medicine is deficient in and resistant to examining vitamin and mineral levels, wait until you ask to test fatty acid levels. The reason is simple: Interpreting fatty-acid levels involves considerably more biochemical knowledge than most doctors have. *Fatty-acid deficiency is one of the major reasons why some folks will never get better.* Know, too, that if you do not look for fatty-acid deficiency, you will not find it.

Sometimes folks naively think that, because their doctor ordered a battery of blood tests, that everything that is wrong with them will show up on those tests. Wrong. Tests only reveal what you are smart enough to look for. The tests usually done with a physical are lumped into one test called a profile, which examines gross indicators of liver, kidney, and bone function as well as advanced diabetes. A profile rarely provides an early indicator of disease before there are symptoms, whereas a fatty-acid test can offer so much more, even to the point of aborting disease long before symptoms appear.

The bottom line here is that the standard chemical profile test is quite rudimentary. It's neither a subtle test nor an early indicator of damage.

Certainly as well, medicine does not generally look for causes of symptoms when they first appear and are easier to correct. Instead, doctors medicate symptoms until they get worse, when more invasive, expensive, and dangerous sorts of treatment come to the fore. On the other hand, testing mineral and fatty-acid levels, for example, can be more subtle and earlier indicators of abnormal chemistry, so those abnormalities can be corrected before a definable disease emerges. It goes without saying that, in the absense of such tests, many folks will remain at a standstill with their diseases simply because no one has taken the time to find out how their bodily chemistry has gone awry. Again, a major cause of symptoms is the slow insidious accumulation of deficiencies, mainly through nutrient loss during the body's work of detoxifying our daily environmental exposures.

Human cells are very complex, and there are many types, all with their own separate functions. For example, a bone cell metabolizes calcium entirely differently from the way a skin cell does. Most cells have unique functions as well. The stomach parietal cell, for example, is the only cell that makes intrinsic factor needed to absorb vitamin B_{12}. How do cells carry on all this complicated and highly unique chemistry? And then how do they harmonize their individual functions with all the other cell types? This truly amazing orchestration is mediated in part by the envelope that surrounds every cell, the cell membrane. You might say it functions as the computer keyboard.

Because the cell membrane is so crucial a determinant of health, I'd better tell you more about it. First off, it is composed mainly of fat. Those fat cravings of yours have a purpose; it is just that we often choose the wrong types of fat to satisfy our urges. Because fat (also called lipid) repels water, fat enables the cell membrane to keep its contents from spilling out and mixing with the rest of the blood. But just as important as its role in keeping the cell self-contained, the membrane also makes and emits many types of messenger molecules that help it orchestrate or integrate with the functions of all the other types of cells.

As a matter of fact, the structure of the membrane is a lot like a sandwich, a lipid sandwich. Only this sandwich has an extremely precise balance of the layers of fatty acids and other nutrients. If such acids and nutrients are deranged in any way, the messenger proteins synthesized and sent out to interact with the rest of the body communicate dangerous messages that precipitate symptoms. If we eat too many trans fatty acids, for example, the cell membrane suffers and aging and disease come all too swiftly.

Clearly, we are the first generation in history to actually change or distort the types and amounts of fats in our cell membranes. As a result, our bodies can malfunction in an unprecedented number of ways and there is a high rate of unwellness. In fact, new diseases are emerging all the time.

How do we slowly accumulate the destructive fatty acids over the years? Diets containing margarine, hydrogenated soybean oil, grocery-store polyunsaturated salad and cooking oils, shortening in baked and other goods, and fried and processed foods are the major culprits. They all help to insidiously damage cell membranes, mimicking all kinds of diseases, including premature aging and cancer as the damage deepens. With this tiny amount of molecular biochemistry, it should be no surprise that some ulcers, for instance, never heal until the bad fatty acids are replaced with the good ones (Das). In other words, many folks will never heal their illness, whether ulcers, gastritis, colitis, IBS, or cancer, until they have given their membranes an oil change. But before you can put the correct amounts of specific oils back in the lipid membrane, you need to know which ones are too high and which are too low.

The fatty-acid test measures thirty essential fatty acids, including the damaging trans fatty acids. When industrial food processors expose oils to high temperatures, they do so to help give the foods they market longer shelflives. High temperature processing, however, twists oil molecules into trans fatty acids. Margarines are as much as 35 percent trans fatty acids.

All hydrogenated oils, soybean and safflower oils, shortenings, fake butters or margarines, and the many baked, fried, and processed foods like bottled salad dressings, cookies, crackers, breads, cereals, and candies contain high amounts of trans fatty acids. Avoid them or eat them very sparingly! Trans fatty acids definitely contribute to our high rate of cardiac disease, cancer, and ill health. They damage cell membranes by displacing the good fatty acids that the body requires in its overall orchestration of the intricate biochemistry of health.

For the fatty-acid test get a prescription, call for the kit, and have your blood drawn at any local lab. The test shows which fatty acids are low and which are high. A physician with special training in fatty-acid chemistry, of course, will prescribe a better regimen for you than a physician who does not. Know that test results are interpreted (although not tailored as well to the individual) for physicians without this expertise.

Table 15 gives a brief synopsis of the paremeters measured by a CDSA, what they most often indicate, and what are some of the common initial remedies to correct them.

Table 15. Simplified Overview of CDSA

CDSA measurement	Most common indications	Starting remedies
Undigested fiber	Poor pancreas, low acid Poor chewing, low bile salts	Take pancreatic enzymes (like Bio-Gest) Increase chewing
Low chymotrypsin	Low secretions as above, bad diet of processed foods, low thyroid, nutrient deficiencies, intestinal blockage	Take pancreatic enzymes (like Bio-Gest), increase chewing, eat brown rice and steamed veggies, get a thorough medical work-up to determine other causes for it
High chymotrypsin	Bad bugs, low stomach acid, high-meat diet, sluggish bowel	Add chymotrypsin Bio-Zyme of Inflazyme Forte, probiotics, herbal antibiotics, natural antibiotics, betaine HCl, low or no-meat diet, fiber and whole grains, greens, and beans
High pH (alkaline)	Poor bugs, low acid, high-meat diet, sluggish bowel	As above
Low pH (acidic)	Bacterial overgrowth, poor pancreal function, fast transit, food allergy, celiac disease, chemical overload, poor diet, nutrient deficiencies	Probiotics, herbal antibiotics, natural antibiotics, pancreas
Poor absorption, high cholesterol	Celiac disease, Candida or other organisms, parasites, food allergy, chemical overload (environmental), poor teeth, poor enzymes, bad bugs, medication damage (NSAIDs, leaky gut), abnormal (fast or slow) transit, insufficient water and/or fiber (whole foods)	Gluten-free diet, yeast program, herbal fighters, food allergy diet, environmental controls, juicing, steaming, blending, pancreas, herbal fighters, find cause for meds and use Aloe Gel Caps and DGL, L-glutamine to at least start to heal gut Butyrates, L-glutamine, special intestinal support

Table 15. Simplified Overview of CDSA (*cont.*)

CDSA measurement	Most common indications	Starting remedies
High b-glucuronidation	High-meat diet, bad bugs, chronic inflammation (chemicals, drugs, (chemicals, drugs, infection, colitis, that could	Eat less meat or omit meat entirely from diet, identify and eradicate cause; in meantime boost glucuronidation pathways with 2–3 twice a day of either Ulva Rigida (Carotec) or
High secretory IgA	lead to cancer) Gut working overtime to fight off bad bugs	Calcium-D-Glucarate (Tyler) Kill bugs, support host's nutritional status and heal gut, beginning with L-glutamine
Low sIgA in presence of bad bugs	A very bad sign that gut is not able to rally to fight with first line of defense	Herbal or prescription antibiotics, natural antibiotic boosters, special intestinal support, liver and glandular support, colostrum
Occult blood	Parasites, roughage, bleeding ulcer, hemorrhoids, colitis, Crohn's CUC, cancer	Artecin or Citramesia, soft fiber, special intestinal supports (see all protocols), medical work-up, try using vitamin C and then stopping to see if occult blood disappears
Bad bugs	Bad food choices Bad gut and/or body Antibiotics	Probiotics, herbal yeast-fighters, prescription antifungals, strenthen host resistance
Any fungi, yeasts, molds	Antibiotics and other medications, nutrient deficiencies, damaged gut immune system.	Probiotics, herbal yeast-fighters, prescription antifungals, strenthen host resistance

Table 16. Leaky gut test (intestinal hyperpermeability)

Leaky gut test measurement	Most common indications	Starting remedies
Elevated levels of lactulose or mannitol or both	Inflammed gut due to NSAIDS, other meds, food allergies, chemical overload (environmental), bad bugs, poor digestion, nutrient deficiencies, hormone deficiencies	As per CDSA, plus L-glutamine butyrates, whole foods and other special intestinal support nutrients to begin to heal the gut
Depressed levels of lactulose or mannitol or both	Malabsorption: this is serious and deserves at least 6 months of gluten-free diet regardless of results of other test for gluten	As above. All included for colitis conditions. When the gut is this badly damaged, life hangs by a thread; reserve weight is minimal and time is of the essence.

Table 17. Comprehensive parasitology

Findings	Prescribed treatments	Natural solutions
Parasites will be identified as to specific ones	Specific treatments will be suggested on report. Metronidazole, a commonly recommended treatment, quite toxic and often useless, leaving worse and new symptoms later.	Evaluate Artecin or Citromesia first as well as Paragard and others in text, as well as all the things to strengthen the host. For all infection is based on how weak the host is, not how strong the bug is.

Mineral Assays

Mineral interpretations should be done by a physician trained in nutritional biochemistry, for there are many minerals that are not present in the assays that if omitted from a program will cause serious problems. Chromium, calcium, molybdenum, vanadium are a few examples, depending on which company's assay was obtained.

As well, to a novice, potassium deficiencies, for example, could mean that potassium is merely needed, when in fact it is usually a more ominous sign that the potassium channel pumps in the cell membrane are defective due to the wrong fatty acids, lack of phosphatidylcholine, inositol hexanicotinate, alpha tocopherol and the tocotrienols, and other crucial cell membrane nutrients.

Heavy Metal Assays

Heavy metal assays may be obtained alone or in combination with minerals, but a physician trained in this is necessary. First, the source of the mercury, as an example, needs to be found, whether it be dietary fish, house paints, incinerator or pesticide exposure, or amalgams. Then, the total body burden needs to be assessed by using oral or injectable chelating nutrients or drugs to see how readily the body is going to give up the metals to the urine and stool to be excreted.

Sometimes getting rid of the mercury can be as simple as taking a super mercury detox cocktail (MDC) two to three times a day, five days on, five days off, while checking urine at twenty-four-hour intervals to see if it is sufficient to mobilize mercury into the urine at the end of each cycle. This can be repeated for a month or two.

The Mercury Detox Cocktail (phase I) in its simplest form:

- one teaspoon of Ultra Pure Ascorbic Acid (Klaire)
- one scoop of Recancostat (Tyler)
- one Mercury Detox (Tyler)
- one Selenium Cruciferate (Ecologic Formulas)
- one scoop of whey (Jarrow, Thorne, or Wakunaga)
- 600 milligrams Lipoic acid crystals (Ecologic Formulas) or capsules (Metabolic Maintenance, Jarrow, or Carlson)
- one scoop 500 milligrams TMG crystals (Longevity Science)
- Take all of the above with two large glasses of water. Take no other nutrients during these days. Use your regular nutrients on the days off the MDC.

One caution with heavy metals: Often there is a small elevation—nothing striking—of two to three metals. The inclination among untrained physicians is to call this normal. However, when you tally up the total toxins the picture is quite different. Be sure all the metals are tallied. You do not want anything more in your body than what belongs there.

Fatty Acids

Fatty-acid assays likewise require expertise. However, if you are simply low in omega-3 oils, and low in EPA and DHA, your cheapest, cleanest, most mercury-free, and best fix that's closest to nature is a teaspoon of cod liver oil (Carlson) a day, or Eskimo-3 Caps (Tyler) if you hate oil. However I like to stay close to nature. You can get away with a tablespoonful two to three times a week if that helps you tolerate it. If you do not tolerate fish, flax oil (organic, dated, refrigerated in health food store, Spectrum, Erasmus brands).

If you have a dihomogammalinolenic acid (DLGA) deficiency, you could start taking Efamol's Evening Primrose Oil (Emerson Ecologics), two capsules, twice a day. Other than that, I would get help and remember that one of the worst things to happen with fatty acids (or any correction) is when the physician follows up on the *balance*. If you get better for a while and then deteriorate again, you passed the mark and everyone missed it.

Food Allergy Tests

It is obvious to avoid the foods that show up on the blood test to determine if they cause symptoms. But you must also remember to avoid other foods in the same botanical family, which may cause even worse symptoms (all in *The E.I. Syndrome, Revised*). For example, if wheat is a potential problem, then oats or rye may be also. Likewise for beef and dairy.

Another excellent lab is MetaMetrix Clinical Laboratory and they offer the following tests:

IgG4 and IgE Food Antibody Assays (Food Antibody Panel)

Sometimes folks are too busy to do a diagnostic diet (described in Chapter 2) to discover their hidden food allergies. And it is particularly stressful to do with some children. Although not as thorough, a blood test can easily determine if you make antibodies to certain foods.

Get a prescription, call the lab to order the kit, take the kit to the blood-drawing lab of your choice. It not only looks at whether or not you make antibodies to any of ninety commonly eaten foods, but how much antibody you make. The limits of food allergy testing via blood tests are that the body has a dozen ways of reacting to a particular kind of food, and this only measures two of them. So just because a food comes up negative does not absolutely mean that it is safe. For example, coffee and alcohol can cause relentless gastritis, but you won't necessarily make antibodies to them.

Likewise, there are false positives, as some folks have a positive test result showing they make antibodies to a food, but when they eat that food they do not notice any symptoms. We make antibodies to things that may have no target organ in the body. For example, the test can be positive because you make antibodies to milk, but nothing happens to you when you drink it. On the flip side, those antibodies could lie down in the pancreas and precipitate diabetes as they have in children. Juvenile diabetics have a high incidence of antibodies against milk, and these antibodies presumably seek out and damage the pancreas or insulin receptors, leading to diabetes.

So how do you interpret the results of food allergy testing? Avoid all the positives for two to four weeks and evaluate your symptoms. If you are not better, it may be because you did not react (false negatives) to foods that do trigger your gut symptoms. In this case you will need to do the diagnostic diet to find the culprits. Then once you have reduced your symptoms, you can slowly add back some of the positives that you hope you now tolerate, adding only one food a day. Not only can some of them be false positives, but as the gut heals, food allergies tend to melt away to varying degrees, depending on the individual and their total load.

Elemental Analysis on Erythrocytes

This test measures the rbc minerals and heavy metals. Arsenic, cadmium, lead, mercury, aluminum, antimony, barium, beryllium, bismuth, boron, lithium, nickel, strontium, and thallium are the heavy metals. The minerals included are copper, chromium, magnesium, manganese, molybdenum, potassium, selenium, sodium, vanadium, and zinc. I find their aluminum and chromium very useful.

Fatty Acid Panel

This is their comprehensive fatty-acid test. The amounts and ratios of fatty acids play a pivotal role in controlling inflammatory reactions. This test measures the essential fatty acids, including the trans fatty acids. Get a prescription, call for the kit, and have blood drawn at a local lab.

Vitamin Panel

They have an abbreviated vitamin panel of vitamins A, E (d-alpha tocopherol), and beta-carotene. You would use this when you want to save money and screen for levels of only three of the main protective antioxidant vitamins.

Candida Antibodies

Measures antibody level to Candida in the blood. A simple blood test is all that is required. It is particularly useful when the titer (antibody level) is changing, which helps you monitor the success of your therapy.

Organic Acids

Remember the organic acid example in the preceding chapter. Organic acids measured in the urine were used to back up the suspicion that an overgrowth of yeast was present and a probable cause of symptoms even though no yeast grew on other tests, because this test can measure telltale chemicals produced by unwanted bugs. It stands to reason they cannot be present in significant enough numbers to cause symptoms, without making substances that prove their existence. Every organism living in the gut has to live, breathe, eat, and produce waste. So if the bugs are present in large enough amounts, their metabolites will leak into the bloodstream and be excreted in the urine.

If you suspect you have yeast overgrowth in the gut, but no test shows it, this test may save the day. This unusual test is easily done and provides information not obtained with other tests. Once you get the prescription and kit, it is a simple urine test you do at home. It measures forty metabolites; some indicate whether there is intestinal dysbiosis or an imbalance in the gut's abnormal amounts of unwanted bugs. Not all of the acids measured are produced by bugs in the gut. Some of the acids suggest a deficiency of various nutrients, while others suggest blocks in important pathways that regulate energy production. There is an interpretive guide that accompanies the test for physicians who are not well versed in the biochemistry of the body.

It can be very frustrating for a person who suspects they have yeast overgrowth in the gut, but cannot convince their physician to treat them for it. Every time they eat sweets or even fruits, they get gas, bloating, indigestion, and even fatigue and brain fog. They have tried all the nonprescription remedies and would like a prescription one, but the stool yeast cultures are negative, so the doctor is hard-pressed to prescribe for a bug they cannot prove exists. The urinary organic acids can save the day.

For example, if there is suspected yeast overgrowth that does not show up on culture, elevated urinary metabolites (chemicals that yeasts throw off into the bloodstream when they are growing) like citromalate, B-ketoglutarate, tartrate, and arabinose suggest there is overgrowth of yeasts (Bernard, Roboz). In fact, it is most important to get rid of these metabolites, or at least reduce their levels, because arabinose forms cross-linked proteins called pentosidines (or pentoses) that accumulate in brain-damaging conditions like Alzheimer's disease (Sell).

Another example of the usefulness of organic acids is in establishing the diagnosis of celiac disease. There are folks for whom the antigliadin and antigluten antibody blood tests (done as standard blood tests) are negative, but who know they have celiac disease because the gut does not heal (assessed by fewer symptoms and/or cessation of weight loss) until they are off all gluten-containing foods, like wheat, rye, oats, and barley. A high excretion of p-cresol, tyrosine, and phenylalanine suggest the presence of celiac, as these metabolites have been found in high amounts in nearly all celiac patients (Van der Heiden, Tamm).

Other toxic metabolites that indicate bacterial or protozoal overgrowth are mapped out by the lab and included in the report for ease of interpretation.

Serum Multiple Analytes Chemistry (SMAC)

This is a forty-one-element assay of liver, kidney, thyroid, bone, iron, and more for general assessment.

Candida Antibodies

These are useful, as discussed, especially if the titer is going up. That is a sure sign of active infection.

Doctor's Data is a third lab for some of these tests:

Minerals: Red Blood Cell and Whole Blood

Doctor's Data offers rbc minerals as well as whole blood minerals. It is important to get both in some circumstances because the body compartmentalizes minerals where it perceives they are best needed. So if you know something is wrong, but the rbc minerals look pretty good, check the whole blood minerals (or vice versa), because the results can be surprisingly diverse. For example, you can look like you have great levels of selenium in the red blood cell, but the levels can be dangerously low in whole blood, inhibiting healing of the gut indefinitely. Always believe the level that is not normal, for the body is continually robbing Peter to pay Paul. It will continually play musical chairs with nutrients that are deficient in the attempt to shuttle them to where they are most needed at a particular moment.

Amino Acids

Amino acids are the building blocks needed for all tissue repair. But they have other uses when the levels of specific ones are abnormal. For example, a high blood level of the amino acid called homocysteine can indicate increased risk of early heart attack, unless corrected with extra folic acid, B_{12}, and betaine. Likewise, this amino acid has been found to be abnormally elevated in folks with IBS (the catch-all term), colitis, Crohn's, enteritis, and other conditions (Cattaneo).

This test is especially important in cases of malabsorption. If the amino acids are low in urine as well as in blood, it is time for serious hyperalimentation. You recall this is where the gut is so damaged that the individual must put it to rest and be fed intravenously (Chapter 6 in the nutrients protocol). Or if this is not possible, they can at least use more easily digestible aids like hydrolyzed Sea Cure and/or UltraClear or UltraInflamX and most likely the celiac diet while a workup including every test in this book is done.

Fecal Toxic Elements

Fecal Toxic Elements looks for toxic excretion of fifteen elements, including mercury, aluminum, cadmium, antimony, and arsenic. These are common contaminants in the body due to foods, medications, auto exhaust, pesticides, dental amalgams, and more. Too many unsuspected toxic elements in the stool can retard healing of the gut indefinitely. The test results indicate if the levels are higher than those found in the normal population. However, I would caution that there are very few folks left with no levels of toxic elements or heavy metals. And as the world becomes progressively more polluted, the "norm" for total toxics goes up. In reality you do not want any toxic elements in your body. Let's look at the fourth lab.

ImmunoSciences Lab offers specialty tests for antibodies against just about anything you need. In addition to antibodies against *H. pylori* and Candida, it has extremely useful antibodies showing sensitivity to environmental chemicals. Remember, chemical sensitivity can be caused by untreated IBS that has caused leaky gut and damaged the chemical detoxification pathways that line the gut and vice versa.

Conversely, chemical sensitivity can be a strong factor that inhibits you from ever getting well. For just like heavy metals, other environmental chemicals can severely damage enzymes and other regulatory proteins. For example, formaldehyde in carpets, mattresses, and other furnishings and construction materials; plastics (phthalic anhydride, trimellitic anhydride, toluene di-isocyanate) that leach into your bottled water or sodas from their containers; glutaraldehyde from dental glues; silicone from breast and other implants; and benzene derivatives in air fresheners are all carcinogens that the body also makes antibodies against in an attempt to protect itself. These can be measured by this unique lab. Levels above norm indicate this may be what is keeping the body from totally healing.

Although the catalog is much more extensive than I have room to devote to it here, let me give you some more pertinent examples of the unique offerings. Sometimes folks have read enough to know they must have Candida overgrowth in their guts. With book in hand supporting them with evidence, they go to their physician, who has no training in environmental medicine, and convince him to prescribe Nystatin. When they start dramatically clearing mysterious symptoms that he had been unsuccessfully trying to help them with for years, he is not opposed to prescribing more for them. And since they are treating themselves without full physician guidance, some of the things they should be doing on order to get completely well are not done.

As a result, every time they try to go off Nystatin their symptoms resurface. So they end up on Nystatin for years. This can trigger the overgrowth of a different kind of Candida, Nystatin-resistant *Candida tropicalis,* which is also very hard to prove on culture tests. Fortunately, this lab has a blood-antibody test for this specific species. For once you know that the body is making abnormal amounts of antibodies against this particular species of yeast, then the appropriate treatment measures can be started, beginning with items outlined in Chapter 3.

As another example, Candida antibodies can cross react with human tissues (Vojdani). In other words, once the body starts trying to protect itself against Candida overgrowth in the gut and leakage of Candida across the leaky gut wall into the bloodstream, it makes antibodies. Unfortunately, some parts of human tissues can resemble parts of the wall of Candida. So these antibodies attack the host's (your!) tissues. Your own antibodies are mistakenly attacking your own organs, trying to destroy them. This is how autoimmune diseases like lupus, rheumatoid arthritis, multiple sclerosis, and thyroiditis begin. The proper treatment (which is beyond the scope of this book) begins with the proper diagnosis. Suffice it to say, any physician interested in top-line diagnostic work that is eons ahead of what "modern" medicine is capable of, should be well versed in what this one-of-a-kind, excellent-quality lab has to offer.

American Environmental Health Foundation

These folks will test your daily drinking water. It does not require a prescription from a physician. Call for price and information about sending a sample of your water for analysis for undesirable contaminants that retard health. The quality of water is taken for granted, but unfortunately it is often quite substandard and can be a source of bacterial contaminants as well as pesticides and other chemicals that hold you back from healing.

Table 18. Summary of Laboratory Tests and Laboratories

Laboratory	Gut Tests	Mineral Tests	Others
Great Smokies	CDSA, Purged parasites, Leaky gut test, Candida Culture	Rbc minerals and heavy metals	H. pylori antibodies, Essential fatty acids, Vitamins, Candida antibodies, Food allergy panel, Amino acids
MetaMetrix		Rbc minerals, Whole blood minerals	Organic acids, IgG4 and IgE food anti-bodies, Candida anti-bodies, SMAC, Amino acids, Vitamins
Doctor's Data		Rbc minerals, Whole blood minerals	Amino acids, Fecal toxic elements, Candida Antibodies
Immunosciences Lab			H. pylori antibodies, Special Candida anti-bodies that are not offered elsewhere, Anti-bodies against environ-mental chemicals, and much more
American Environmental Health Foundation			Tests drinking water for chemical and biological contaminants

Simplifying the Solutions

What test you may need really depends on the problem itself, especially if it defies cause or cure. On the other hand, if you can self-diagnose your problem and, by following the suggestions described throughout this book, begin your own cure, then you may not need tests at all. For instance, if you have simple aggravating indigestion because of a diet high in processed foods, a monotonous diet of the same foods (antigens), or stressful eating conditions, you could take action by changing your eating habits with meals of one, two, or three whole, yet different, foods taken quietly and slowly. At the same time, and to help quicken the pace of your cure, you could add in Rhizinate before meals and a simple digestive enzyme after meals.

If you have just concluded an antibiotic regimen for sinusitis, prostate or bladder infections, or if your symptoms worsen whenever eating sweets or ferments—and you now suspect that Candida overgrowth caused your chronic indigestion—the same kinds of measures as mentioned above can be taken here.

In fact, folks have completely healed themselves of Candida overgrowth with a diet of fresh vegetables (steamed and raw), limited amounts of starchy carbohydrates like sweet squashes and potatoes, and no sweets or ferments. If you are a carnivore, of course, you would concentrate on what meats you eat and how best to select them to secure relief. Other folks need only add one or another nonprescription remedy for a few weeks to feel healthy again.

Should your new diet, stress reduction, or nonprescription remedies help you, but symptoms still remain, then you have numerous options ahead of you. Just choose one, follow it, and see if it works. If it doesn't, change course. No course of treatment is cast in stone.

Certainly, if a logical first step involves a medical diagnosis, then start with the CDSA. Alternatively, if you have limited funds or are enrolled in a medical program that does not cover tests, just do the 7-Day Candida Culture.

Clearly, a medical diagnosis will help to cinch which of the more powerful prescription treatments you should be on. If you already have a diagnosis, on the other hand, and you failed to improve sufficiently by following the regimen prescribed for you, you might want to check your mineral and fatty-acid levels. Or you could turn to the many fine physicians trained in environmental medicine and nutritional biochemistry to help you pinpoint why you don't feel completely well.

Whatever route you decide to take, after reading and rereading this book you will do so armed with the knowledge that you need not be a victim of medicine's traditional reliance on drugs; that alone, or with your doctor, you will be able to begin healing yourself.

A New You

You have crossed the Rubicon. With the new knowledge and perspectives on healing, self-healing, and medically aided healing you have learned from this book, you will begin to live anew. By taking control of your health, you should be able to enjoy your life to its fullest potential. By learning how to avoid the dangers posed by traditional medicine and how to make medicine work best for you, you have opened a door unto yourself and onto the world, where you can live with a vitality and purpose you may never have felt before.

Before we close, let's take a few giant steps back with a few handy tear-out sheets you might want to post on your refrigerator door for easy quick reference.

Reminders of aids to be used alone or in combinations

For *emergency* stomach aid after a night of overindulgence that causes heartburn, indigestion, acid reflux:

Gastro-Relief or Rhizinate or Gastromet
Aloe Gel Caps (equivalent to one cup juice)
Similase or Pancreatin or Bio-Gest
Oil of Oregano
Ginger tea or GingerMax
Pepto Bismol
Elevate the head legs of the bed (don't just prop your chest, but your
    whole torso to avoid reflux)

For ongoing lower cramps, bloating, indigestion, constipation, or alternating diarrhea:

Similase or Pancreatin or Bio-Gest
Paragard
Kyolic, Kyo-Green, Kyo-Dophilus
Pure Body Program
Arcetin or Citramesia
L-Glutamine

Never lose sight of the simple little things:

And lest you become too enamored with the world of medicine, never forget common sense and the basics. Perhaps these tips alongside your emergency stomach remedies would serve as a helpful reminder, for even if you accomplish half of them, you are half way to a healthier gut:

Twelve quick tips for a healthier gut

- Avoid eating and drinking two to three hours before bed
- Have smaller meals at night
- Do not lie down after meals
- Eat comfortably seated in a relaxed atmosphere with pleasant company and conversation
- Don't wear tight clothing to the table
- Don't dilute your digestive juices with drinks
- Avoid alcohol or limit yourself to one to two glasses of wine
- Chew each mouthful until it is liquid
- Eat at least 85 percent of foods in their whole or near-whole state, not ground into pasty flours, overcooked, and processed
- Drink at least a half gallon of water (two quarts) a day between meals

- Avoid antibiotics when other options are available
- Limit white flour, white sugar, and trans fatty acids (fried foods and processed foods with hydrogenated soy and other vegetable oils, margarines), as these are the worst gut-damaging culprits

With a healthier gut, you'll be able to tolerate an occasional indiscretionary evening with friends without paying for it later.

Healing from the Inside Out

In closing, you now have at your disposal the most complete, up-to-date approach available for folks with an ailing gut. Don't be overwhelmed by the amount of information here. You have just had a course at the medical school of the future where cause, not a handful of drugs, is the concern. So you need to be exposed to the gamut of possible causes.

Fortunately for you this course has been streamlined for you to look at merely the 80/20 rule of causes and cures. Otherwise, it would have been four times larger. For 80 percent of folks will get well with using only 20 percent of what we have available.

So start easy with a simple diet change or elimination of a probable culprit, then try a remedy or two for what you have deduced you have. With what you have learned here, chances are you will be right. You can only grow with your knowledge base, so come back to different sections from time to time and see what you have been avoiding doing that now seems appropriate for you.

Never lose sight of the fact that even a seemingly innocent-sounding symptom like constipation can result in serious consequences, like autoimmune diseases, or the less severe but enormously annoying pain, surgery, and recurrence of anal tears, fissures, and fistulas. Yet all conditions have been completely cured in many folks simply by eliminating cow's milk from the diet (Iacono). Likewise potentially fatal ulcerative colitis has markedly improved in some with mere cod liver oil (Stenson). On the flip side, medicine is so frustrated now that they have resorted to more cancer-causing chemotherapy drugs to quell serious colitis (Stotland), and all because they do not look for the causes you have learned about here.

Furthermore, the gut is not an isolated organ. It makes protein messengers (vasoactive intestinal peptides) that turn on brain moods or allergic symptoms in the nose (Mosimann). The gut talks to the rest of the body and the body talks to the gut. And since half of the body's immune system as well as its detoxification resides in the walls of the gut, your capability of healing anything from depression to cancer depends on the health of the gut.

You should never have another perplexing or incurable gut symptom again, now that you are well versed in gut level medicine. And the rest of your health should prosper as well, since the road to health is paved with good intestines.

No, there is no going back from this stage. You are a new person who has learned that every symptom has a cause and cure, most of which can be pretty logical and simple. And best of all, most are within your grasp. You are now captain of your ship, master of control, champion of your gut.

References

Introduction

Cohen S, Parkman HP. Heartburn—a serious symptom (editorial). *New Engl J Med* 1999; 340: 878–879.

Kuipers EJ, Lundell L, Klinkenberg-Knol EC, et al. Atrophic gastritis and *Helicobacter pylori* infection in patients with reflux esophagitis treated with omeprazole or fundoplication. *N Eng J Med* 1996:334:1018–1022.

Lagergren J, Bergstrom R, Lingren A, Nyren O. Symptomatic gastroesophageal reflux as a risk factor for esophageal adenocarcinoma. *New Engl J Med* 1999;340:825–831.

Stotland BR, Cirigliano MD, Lichtenstein GR. Medical therapies for inflammatory bowel disease. *Hospital Practice* May 15, 1998; 141–168.

Zucca A, Bertoni F, Cavalli F, et al. Molecular analysis of the progression from *Helicobacter pylori*-associated chronic gastritis to mucosa-associated lymphoid-tissue lymphoma on the stomach. *New Engl J Med* 1998; 338(12): 803–810.

Chapter 1

Allen FE. One man's suffering spurs doctors to probe pesticide-drug link. *Wall Street Journal*. A1, October 14, 1991.

Arky R. *Physicians' Desk Reference,* 53rd ed. Montvale, NJ: Medical Economics Co., 1999.

Arky R. *Physicians' Desk Reference for Nonprescription Drugs,* 19th ed. Montvale, NJ: Medical Economics Co., 1998.

Banks WA, et al. Aluminum increases permeability for the blood-brain barrier to labeled DSIP and beta-endorphin: possible implications for senile and dialysis dementias. *Lancet* 1983; 26:1227–1279.

Cannon LA, Heiselman DE, Dougherty JM, Jones J. Magnesium levels in cardiac arrest victims: Relationship between magnesium levels and successful resuscitation. *Ann Emerg Med* 1987; 16:1195–1198.

Cox I, Campbell M, Dowson D. Red blood cell magnesium and chronic fatigue syndrome. *Lancet* 1991; 227:757–760.

Darchy B, Le Miere E, Domart Y, et al. Iatrogenic diseases as a reason for admission to the intensive care unit. *Arch Intern Med* 1999;159:71–78.

Drossman DA, Li Z, Andruzzi E, Shiming L, et al. U.S. householder survey of functional gastrointestinal disorders, prevalence, sociodemography, and health impact. *Dig Dis Sci* 1993;38:1569–1580.

Eisenberg DM, Kessler RC, Delbanco TL, et al. Unconventional medicine in the United States. *New Engl J Med* 1993;328:246–252.

Erickson. Mortality in selected cities with fluoridated and non-fluoridated water supplies. *New Engl J Med* 1978; 298:1112–1116.

Fitzpatrick AL., Daling JR, Weissfelf JL, et al. Use of calcium-channel blockers and breast carcinoma risk in postmenopausal women. *Cancer* 1997; 80:1438–1447.

Galbraith RA, Michnovicz. The effects of cimetidine on the oxidative metabolism of estradiol. *New Engl J Med* 1989;321:269–274.

Heckbert SR, Longstreth WT, Rufberg CD, et al. The association of antihypertensive agents with MRI white matter findings and with modified mini-mental state examination in older adults. *J Amer Geriatric Soc* 1997; 45:1423–1433.

Jones R, Lydeard S. Prevalence of symptoms of dyspepsia in the community. *Brit Med J* 1989;298:30–32.

Johannessen T, Petersen H, Klevell PM, et al. The predictive value of history in dyspepsia. *Scand J Gastroenterol* 1990;25:689–697.

Kaehny WD, et al. Gastrointestinal absorption of aluminum from aluminum-containing antacids. *New Engl J Med* 1977;296:1389–1390.

Kohn PD. A brief report on the association of drinking water fluoridation and the incidence of osteo sarcoma among young males. *New Jersey Dept of Health* Nov. 8, 1992.

Lazarou J, Pomeranz BH, Core PN. Incidence of adverse drug reactions in hospitalized patients. *J Amer Med Assoc* 1998;279:1200–1205.

Lieber CS. *J Amer Med Assoc* 1990.

Mitchell CM, Drossman DA. Survey of the AGA membership relating to patients with functional gastrointestinal disorders. *Gastroenterology* 1987;92:1282–1284.

Motoyama T, Sano H, Fukuzaki H. Oral magnesium supplementation in patients with essential hypertension. *Hypertension* 1989, 13:227–232.

Perl DP, Brody AR. Detection of aluminum by semi-x-ray spectrometry with neurofibrillary tangle-bearing neurons of Alzheimer's disease. *Neurotox* 1990: 133–137.

Perl DP, Brody AR. Alzheimer's disease: x-ray spectro-metric evidence of aluminum accumulation in neurofibrillary bearing neurons. *Sci* 1980:297–299.

Rogers SA. Unrecognized magnesium deficiency masquerades as diverse symptoms: Evaluation of an oral magnesium challenge test. *Internat Clin Nutr Rev* 1991;11;3:117–125.

Shamsuddin AM. *IP6, Nature's Revolutionary Cancer-Fighter.* New York: Kensington Books, 1998.

Chapter 2

Bentley SJ, et al. Food hypersensitivity in irritable bowel syndrome. *Lancet* 1983;II:295–297.

Johansson SG, Dannaeus A, Liya G. The relevance of anti-food antibodies for the diagnosis of food allergy. *Ann Allergy* 1984;53:665–672.

Jones VA, Shorthouse M, Hunter JO, et al. Food intolerance: a major factor in the pathogenesis of irritable bowel syndrome. *Lancet* 1982;:1115–1117.

Gledhill T, et al. Epidemic hypochlorhydria. *Brit J Med* 1985;289: 383–386.

Hyams JS. Sorbitol intolerance: an unappreciated cause of functional gastrointestinal complaints. *Gastroenterology* 1983;84: 30–33.

Kozlovsky AS, et al. Effects of diets high in simple sugars on urinary chromium losses. *Metabolism* 1986;35;515–518.

Lawrie, et al. The urinary excretion of bacterial amino-acid metabolites by rats fed saccharin in the diet. *Food Chem Toxicol* 1985;23:445–450.

Phelan JJ, et al. Celiac disease: the abolition of gliadin toxicity by enzymes from *Aspergillus niger. Clin Sci Molec Med* 1977;53:35–43.

Ravich WJ, et al. Fructose: incomplete intestinal absorption in humans. *Gastroenterology* 1989;92:383–389.

Rogers SA. *Depression Cured At Last!* Syracuse, NY: Prestige Publishing, 1997.

White R, Jobling S, Parker MG, et al. Environmentally persistent alkylphenolic compounds are estrogenic. *Endocrinology* 1994;135:175–182.

Zwetchkenbaum JF, Burkoff R. The irritable bowel syndrome and hypersensitivity. *Ann Allergy* 1988;60:1–3.

References on Vanadium

Bhanoit S, McNeill JH. Vanadyl sulfate lowers plasma insulin and blood pressure in spontaneously hypertensive rats. *Hypertension* 1993;24;625–632.

McNeill JH, Yuen VG, et al. Bis(maltolato)oxovanadium (IV) is a potent insulin mimic. *J Med Chem* 1992;35;1489–1491.

Verma S, Cam MC, McNeill JH. Nutritional factors that can favorably influence the glucose/insulin system: Vanadium. *J Am Coll Nutr* 1998;17;1:11–18.

References on Olestra

Jones DY, Miller KW, Koonsvitsky, et al. Serum 25-hydroxyvitamin D concentrations of free-living subjects consuming olestra. *Amer J Clin Nutr* 1991;53(5):1281–1287.

Lafranconi WM, Long PH, Atkinson JEA, Knezivich AL, Wooding WL. Chronic toxicity and carcinogenicity of olestra in Swiss CD-1 mice. *Food Chem Toxicol* 1994;32(9):789–798.

Miller KW, Wood FE, Stuard SB, Alden CL. A 20-month olestra feeding study in dogs. *Food Chem Toxicol* 1991;29(7):427–435.

References on MSG

Blaylock RL. *Excitotoxins: The Taste That Kills.* Santa Fe, NM: Health Press, 1994.

Reif-Lehrer L, Stemmerman, MG. Monosodium glutamate intolerance in children. *N Engl J Med* 1975;293:1204–1205.

References on Aspartame

Blundell JE, Hill AJ. Paradoxical effects of an intense sweetener (aspartame) on appetite. *Lancet* 1986;I:1092–1093.

Roberts HJ. Reactions attributed to aspartame-containing products: 551 cases. *J Appl Nutr* 1988; 40:85–94.

Roberts HJ. Aspartame and hyperthyroidism, a presidential affliction reconsidered. *Townsend Letter for Doctors & Patients*, 86–87, May 1997.

References on Saccharin

Drenowski A. Intense sweeteners and the control of appetite. *Nutr Rev* 1995;53 (1):1–7.

Rogers PJ, Blundell JE. Separating the actions of sweetness and calories: effects of saccharin and carbohydrates on hunger and food intake in human subjects. *Physiol Behav* 1989;45:1093–1099.

References on Additives

Cort WM. Effects of treatment with food additives on nutrients. Karmas E, Harris RS, eds. In *Nutritional Evaluation of Food Processing*, 3rd ed. New York: Van Nostrand Reinhold, 1988.

Dwivedi BK, Arnold RG. Chemistry of thiamin degradation in food products and model system: a review. *J Agric Food Chem* 1973;21:54–60.

Moneret-Vautian DA, Kanny G. Food and drug additives: hypersensitive and intolerance. In *Human Toxicology* Descotes, J, ed. New York: Elsevier Science B.V., 1996.

Schroeder HA. Losses of vitamins and trace minerals resulting from processing and preservation of foods. *Am J Clin Nutr* 19:24;562–573, 1971.

References on Sugar

Bethea MC. *Sugar Busters—Cut Sugar To Trim Fat*. New York: Ballantine Books, 1998.

Dufty W. *Sugar Blues*. Denver: Nutri-Books, 1975.

Gottschall E. *Breaking the Vicious Cycle*. Kirkton, Ontario: Kirkton Press, 1994.

Appleton N. *Lick the Sugar Habit*. Garden City Park, NY: Avery Publishers, 1996.

Hurst AF, Knott FA. Intestinal carbohydrate dyspepsia. *Quart J Med* 1930; 24;171–180.

Preuss HG, Zein M, Knapka J, et al. Sugar-induced blood pressure elevations over the lifespan of three substrains of Wistar rats. *J Am Coll Nutr* 1998;17(1): 36–47.

Scriver CR, Beaudet AL, Sly WS, Valle D, eds. *The Metabolic Basis of Inherited Disease,* vol. 2. New York: McGraw-Hill, 1989.

Szanto S, Yudkin J. The effect of dietary sucrose on blood lipids, serum insulin, platelet adhesiveness and body weight in human volunteers. *Postgraduate Med J* 1969;45:602–607.

References on Opioid Receptors

Boublik JH, et al. Coffee contains potent opiate receptor binding activity. *Nature* 1983;301:246–248.

Fukodome JS. Opioid peptides derived from wheat gluten: their isolation and characterization. *Febs Lett* 1992;296:107–111.

Karjalainen J, et al. A bovine albumin peptide as a possible trigger of insulin-dependent diabetes mellitus. *New Engl J Med* 1992;327:302–307.

Kurek M, et al. A naturally occurring opioid peptide from cow's milk, beta-casomorphine-7, is a direct histamine releaser in man. *Int Arch Allergy Immunol* 1992;97:115–120.

References on Diet

Brostoff J, Challacombe SJ. *Food Allergy and Intolerance.* Philadelphia: Bailliere Tindall, 1987.

Gallinger S, Rogers SA. *Macro Mellow*, Syracuse, NY: Prestige Publishers, 1992.

Jones VA, et al. Crohn's disease: maintenance of remission by diet. *Lancet* 1985;2:177–80.

Riordan AM, et al. Treatment of active Crohn's disease by exclusion diet: East Anglian multi-center controlled trial. *Lancet* 1993;342:1131–1134.

Rogers, SA. *The E. I. Sydrome,* revised, Syracuse, NY: Prestige Publishers, 1997.

Rowe AH, et al. Regional enteritis: its allergic aspects. *Gastroenterology* 1953;23:554–571.

Chapter 3

Alexander JG. Thrush bowel infection: existence, incidence, prevention and treatment, particularly by a *Lactobacillus acidophilus* preparation. *Curr Med Drugs* 1967;8:3–11.

Baker H, Frank O. Absorption, utilization and clinical effectiveness of allithiamines compared to water soluble thiamines. *J Nutr Sci Vitaminol* 1976;22 (Supp): 63–68.

Bernard EM, Wong B, Armstrong D. Sterioisomeric configuration of arabinitol in serum, urine, and tissues in invasive candidiasis. *J Infect Dis* 1985;151(4): 711–715.

Bolivar R, et al. Candidiasis of the gastrointestinal tract. In Bodey, GP, Fainstein, V, eds. *Candidiasis.* New York: Raven Press, 1985.

Brabander JO, Blank F, Butas CA. Intestinal moniliasis in adults. *Can Med Assoc J* 1957;77:478–482.

Caporaso M, et al. Anti-fungal activity in human urine and serum after ingestion of garlic *(Allium sativum)*. *Antibicrob Agents Chemother* 1983;23(5):700–702.

Caselli M, Trevisani L, Bighi S, et al. Dead fecal yeasts and chronic diarrhea. *Digestion* 1988;41:142–148.

Eaton KK. Sugars in food intolerance and gut fermentation. *J Nutr Med* 1992;3: 295–301.

Eaton KK, McLaren, Howard JMH. Abnormal gut fermentation: laboratory studies reveal deficiency of B vitamins, zinc, and magnesium. *J Nutr Bioch* 1993; 4:636–638.

Eaton KK, Howard MA. Fungal-type dysbiosis of the gut: The occurrence of fungal diseases and the response to challenge with yeasty and mould-containing foods. *J Nutr & Environ Med* 1998;8:247–255.

Gupta TP, Ehrenpreis MN. Candida-associated diarrhea in hospitalized patients. *Gastroent,* 1990;98:780–785.

Hunnusett A, Howard J, Davies S. Gut fermentation (or the "auto-brewery" syndrome): a clinical test with initial observations and discussion. *J Nutr Med* 1990;1:33–38.

Igram C. *The Cure Is in the Cupboard: How to Use Oregano for Better Health.* Buffalo Grove, IL: Knowledge House, 1997.

Iwata K. A review of the literature on drunken symptoms due to yeast in the gastrointestinal tract. In Iwata K, ed. *Yeasts and Yeast-like Microorganisms in Medical Science.* Toyko: University of Tokyo Press, 1976.

Iwata K, et al. Studies on the toxins produced by *Candida albicans* with special reference to their etiopathological role. In Iwata K, ed. *Yeasts and Yeast-like Microorganisms in Medical Science.* Tokyo: University of Tokyo Press, 1976.

Kabe J, et al. Antigenicity of fractions from extracts of *Candida albicans. J Allergy* 1971;47:59–75.

Kaji H, et al. Intragastrointestinal alcohol fermentation syndrome: report of two cases and review of the literature. *J Forensic Sci Soc* 1984;24:461–471.

Kane JG, Chretien JH, Garagusi V. Diarrhea caused by Candida. *Lancet* 1976;335–336.

Moore GS, et al. The fungicidal and fungistatic effects of an aqueous garlic extract on medically important yeast-like fungi. *Mycologia* 1977;69:341–348.

Mutsukawa D, et al. Studies on thiamine deficiency due to bacterial thiaminase, III. Further investigations of thiamine disease. *J Vitaminol* 1965;2:1–14.

Odds FC. Pathogenesis of Candida infections. *J Am Acad Dermatol* 1994;31: S2–S5.

Palma C, et al. Lactoferrin release and interleukin-1, interleukin-6, and tumor necrosis factor production by human polymorphonuclear cells stimulated by various lipopolysaccharides: relationship to growth inhibition of *Candida albicans. Infection Immun* 1992;60;11:4604–46011.

Portelli J, et al. Effect of compounds with antibacterial activities in human milk in respiratory syncytial virus and cytomegalovirus in vitro. *J Med Microbiol* 1998;47(11):1015–1018.

Puddu P, et al. Antiviral effect of bovine lactoferrin saturated with metal ions on early steps of human immunodeficiency virus type I infection. *Internat J Biochem Cell Biol* 1998;30(9):1055–1062.

Ridge JM. The metabolism of acetaldehyde by the brain in vivo. *Biochem J* 1963;80:95–100.

Simonopoulos AP, Coring T, Rerat A, eds. *Intestinal Flora, Immunity, Nutrition and Health, World Review of Nutrition and Dietetices, #74,* NY: Karger, 1993.

Stiles JC, Sparks W, Ronzio RA, The inhibition of *Candida albicans* by oregano. *J Appl Nutr* 1995; 47(4):96–102.

Stephan W, et al. Antibodies from colostrum in oral immunotherapy. *J Clin Chem Clin Biochem* 1990;28(1):19–23.

Tadi PP, et al. Anti-Candida and anti-carcinogenic potentials of garlic. *Int Clin Nutr Rev* 1990;10(4):423–429.

Truss CO. Tissue injury induced by *C. albicans:* mental and neurological manifestations. *J Orthomol Psych* 1980;7:17–37.

Truss CO. Metabolic abnormalities in patients with chronic Candidiasis. The acetaldehyde hypothesis. *J Orthomol Med* 1983;13(2):1–28.

Vojdani A, Rahimian P, Kalhor H, Mordechai E. Immunological cross reactivity between *Candida albicans* and human tissue. *J Clin & Lab Immunol* 1996;48: 1–15.

Zaika LL, Kissinger JC. Inhibitory and stimulatory effects of oregano on *Lactobacillus plantarum* and *Pediococcus cerevisiae*. *J Food Sci* 1981;46: 1205–1210.

Chapter 4

References on H. pylori

Alston TA, Abeles RH. Enzymatic conversion of the antibiotic metronidazole to an analog of thiamine. *Arch Biochem Biophys* 1987;257(2):357–362.

Baker B. *H. pylori* suggested as possible underlying factor in rosacea. *Skin & Allergy News*, page 4, Sept 1994.

Baker ME. Licorice and enzymes other than 11B-hydroxysteroid dehydrogenase: an evolutionary perspective. *Steroids* 1994;59:136–141.

Bardhan, et al. Clinical trial of deglycyrrhized liquorice in gastric ulcer. *Gut* 1978;19:779–782.

Bayerdorffer E, Neubauer A, et al. Regression of primary gastric lymphoma of mucosa-associated lymphoid tissue type after cure of *Helicobacter pylori* infection. *Lancet* 1995;345:1591–1594.

Blaser MJ. The bacteria behind ulcers. *Scientific American*, Feb 1996;104–107.

Boren T, Falk P, Roth KA, et al. Attachment *Helicobacter pylori* to human gastric epithelium mediated by blood group antigens. *Science* 1993;262:1892.

Borody T, Noona T, Cole P, et al. Triple therapy of *C. pylori* can reverse hypochlorhydria. *Am J Gastroenterology* 1989;96:A53.

Calvert R, Randerson J, et al. Genetic abnormalities during transition from *Helicobacter-pylori*-associated gastritis to low-grade MALToma. *Lancet* 1995;345;8941:26–27.

Das SK, Das V, et al. Deglycyrrhizinated licorice in aphthous ulcers, *JAPI* 1989;37(10):647.

Dehpour AR, Zolfaghari ME, Samadian T, Vahedi Y. The protective effect of licorice components and their derivatives against gastric ulcer induced by aspirin in rats. *J Pharm Pharmacol* 1994;46:148–149.

De Koster E, Buset M, Fernandes E, et al. *Helicobacter pylori:* the link with gastric cancer. *Europ J Cancer Prev* 1994;3(3):247–257.

Doll R, Hill ID, et al. Clinical trial of a triterpenoid liquorice compound in gastric and duodenal ulcer. *Lancet* 1962;2;793–796.

Fendrick AM, Chernew ME, Scheiman JM, et al. Clinical and economic effects of population-based *Helicobacter pylori* screening to prevent gastric cancer. *Arch Intern Med* 1999;159:142–148.

Forman D, Newell DDG, Fullerton R, et al. Association between infection with *Helicobacter pylori* and risk of gastric cancer: evidence from a prospective investigation, *Brit Med J* 1991;301:1302–1305.

Fuhrman B, Buch S. Licorice extract and its major polyphenol glabridin protect low-density lipoprotein against lipid peroxidation: in vitro and ex vitro studies in humans and in atherosclerotic apolipoprotein E-deficient mice. *Amer J Clin Nut.* 1997;66:267–275.

Gledhill T, et al. Epidemic hypochlorhydria. *Brit J Med* 1985;289: 383–386.

Glick L. Deglycrrhizinated liquorice in peptic ulcer, *Lancet* 1982;2:817.

Gross H, Freundich N, Dawley H. Is cancer a contagious disease: No. *Business Week*, July 14, 1997:70–76.

Henschel E, Brandstatter G, Dragosics B, et al. Effect of ranitidine and amoxicillin plus metronidazole on the eradication of *Helicobacter pylori* and the recurrence of duodenal ulcer. *New Engl J Med* 1993;328:308–312.

Hood HM, Wark C, Scott MW, et al. Screening for *Helicobacter pylori* and non-steroidal anti-inflammatory drug use in Medicare patients hospitalized with peptic ulcer disease. *Arch Intern Med* 1999;159:149–154.

Horwich L, Galloway R. Treatment of gastric ulceration with carbenoxolone sodium: clinical and radiological evaluation. *Brit Med J* 1965;2:1274–1277.

Hwang H, Dwyer J, Russell RM. Diet, *Helicobacter pylori* infection, food preservation and gastric cancer risk: are there new roles for preventative factors. *Nutr Rev* 1994 52(3):75–83.

Ito M, Sato A, et al. Mechanism of inhibitory effect of glycyrrhizin on replication of human immunodeficiency virus (HIV). *Antivir Res* 1988;10:289–298.

Jancin B. Pushing the *H. pylori* envelope: treat everyone with dyspepsia. *Family Practice News* 1994;1:14.

Kassir ZA. Endoscope controlled trial of four drug regimens in the treatment of chronic duodenal ulceration. *Irish Med J* 1985;78:153–156.

Khuylusi S. The effect of unsaturated fatty acids on *Helicobacter pylori* in vitro. *M Med Micro* 1995;42(4):276–282.

Knipp U, Birkholz S, et al. Immune suppressive effects of *Helicobacter pylori* on human peripheral blood mononuclear cells. *Med Microbiol & Immunol* 1993;182(2):63–76.

Kuipers EJ, Uyterlinde AM, et al. Long-term sequelae of *Helicobacter pylori* gastritis, *Lancet* 1995;345:1525–1528.

Kuipers EJ, Uyterlinde AM, Pena AS, et al. Increase of *Helicobacter pylori*-associated corpus gastritis during acid suppressive therapy: implications for long-term safety. *Am J Gastroenterol* 1995;90:1041–1046.

Lewis JR. Carbenoxolone sodium in the treatment of peptic ulcer. *J Amer Med Assoc* 1974;229:460–461.

Logan RPH, Walker MM, Misiewicz JJ, et al. Changes in the intragastric distribution of *Helicobacter pylori* during treatment with omeprazole. *Gut* 1995;36:12–16.

McColl K, Murray L, El-Omar E, Hilditch T. Symptomatic benefit from eradicating *Helicobacter pylori* infection in patients with nonulcer dypepsia. *New Engl J Med* 1998;339:1869–1874.

Morgan AG, McAdam WAF, et al. Comparison between cimetidine and Caved-S in the treatment of gastric ulceration, and subsequent maintenance therapy. *Gut* 1982;23;5455–5451.

Multicenter Trial. Treatment of duodenal ulcers with glycyrrhinizin acid-reduced liquorice, *Brit Med J* 1973; 773(3):501–503.

Munoz N. Is *Helicobacter pylori* a cause of gastric cancer? An appraisal of the seroepidemiological evidence. *Cancer Epidem Biomarkers & Prev* 1994; 3(5):445–451.

Murray MT. *Natural Alternatives to Over-the-counter and Prescription Drugs.* New York: William Morrow, 1994.

Noach LA, Bertola MA, Schwartz MP, et al. Treatment of *Helicobacter pylori* infection and evaluation of various therapeutic trials. *Europ J Gastroenterol Hepatol* 1994;6:585–591.

Nomura A, Stemmewrmann GN, Blasaer MJ, et al. *Helicobacter pylori* infection and gastric carcinoma among Japanese Americans in Hawaii. *New Engl J Med* 1991;325:1132–1136.

Parsonnet J, Friedman GD, Vandersteen DP, et al. *Helicobacter pylori* infection and the risk of gastric carcinoma. *N Engl J Med* 1991;325:1127–1131.

Pompei R, Flore O, et al. Glycyrrhizic acid inhibits virus growth and inactivates virus particles. *Nature* 1979;281:689–690.

Riccardi VM, Rotter JI, Familial *Helicobacter pylori* infection. *Ann Intern Med* 1994;120:1043–1045.

Slomiany BL, et al. Gastroprotective agents in mucosal defense against *Helicobacter pylori*. *Gen Pharmacol* 1994;25:833–841.

Takeuchi T, Shiratori K, et al. Secretin as a potential mediator of antiulcer actions of mucosal protective agents. *J Clin Gastroenterol* 1991;13 (suppl. 1):583–587.

Tangri KK, Seth PK, et al. Biochemical study of anti-inflammatory and anti-arthritic properties of glycyrrhetic acid. *Biochem Pharmacol* 1965;14: 1277–1281.

Tarnawski A. Prevention and treatment of gastrointestinal mucosal injury with cytoprotective agents. *Med J Australia* 1985;142;(suppl)13–17.

The Eurogast Study Group. An international association between *Helicobacter pylori* infection and gastric cancer. *Lancet* 1993;341:1359.

Turpie AG, Runcie J, et al. Clinical trial of deglycyrrhizinated liquorice in gastric ulcer. *Gut* 1969;10:299–303.

Uemura N, Mukai T, Okamoto W, et al. Effect of *Helicobacter pylori* eradication on subsequent development of cancer after endoscopic resection of early gastric cancer. *Cancer Epidemiol Biomarkers Prev* 1997;6:639–642.

Van Marle J. Deglycyrrhizinised liquorice (DGL) and the renewal of rat stomach epithelium. *Eur J Pharmcol* 1981;72:219–225.

Werbach MR, Murray MT. *Botanical Influences on Illness*. Tarzana, CA: Third Line Press, 1994.

Wotherspoon AC, et al. Regression of primary low-grade B-cell gastric lymphoma of mucosa-associated lymphoid tissue type after eradication of *Helicobacter pylori*. *Lancet* 1993 342(8871):575–577.

Yoshikawa M, Matsui Y, et al. Effects of glycyrrhizin on immune-medicated cytotoxicity. *J Gastroenterol Hepatol* 1997, 12:243–248.

Zucca A, Bertoni F, Cavalli F, et al. Molecular analysis of the progression from *Helicobacter pylori*-associated chronic gastritis to mucosa-associated lymphoid-tissue lymphoma on the stomach. *New Engl J Med* 1998;338(12): 803–810.

References on Other Bad Bugs and Irradication

Kuzin AM, Kryukova LM. Mutagenic action of metabolites formed in irradiated plants. *Dolklady Akad Nauk USSR* 1961;137:205–206.

Leonard RE. Chicken feces fine to eat, says new USDA proposal. *Nutrition Week* 1994;24(27):4–5.

Makinen Y, et al. Cytotoxic effects of extracts from gamma-irradiated pineapples. *Nature* 1967;214: 413.

Piccioni R. Analysis of data on the impact of food processing by ionizing radiation on health and the environment. *Int J Biosoc Res* 1998;9(2):203–212.

References on Paragard Ingredients

Adetumbi M, et al. *Allium sativum* (garlic) inhibits lipid synthesis by *Candida albicans: Antimicrob Agents Chemother* 1986;30:499–501.

Amin AH, et al. Berberine sulfate: antimicrobial activity, bioassay, and mode of action. *Can J Microbiol* 1969;15;1067–1076.

Amonkar SV, Banerji A. Isolation and characterization of larvacidal principle of garlic. *Science* 1972;174:1343–1344.

Bhakat MP, et al. Therapeutic trial of Berberine sulfate in nonspecific gastroenteritis. *Ind Med J* 1974;68:19–23.

Bhargana UC, Westfall BA. Antitumor activity of *Juglans nigra* (black walnut) extractives. *J Pharm Sci* 1968;57;1674–1677.

Choudhry VP, Sabir M, Bhide VN. Berberine in giardiasis. *Indian Pediatr* 1972;9:143–146.

Clark AM, Jurgens TM, Hufford CD. Antimicrobial activity of juglone. *Phytother Res* 1990;4:1–11.

Desai AB, et al. Berberine in treatment of diarrhea. *Indian Pediatr* 1971;8:462–465.

Gupte S. Use of berberine in treatment of giardiasis. *Am J Dis Child* 1975;129:866.

Hahn FE, Ciak J. Berberine. *Antibiotics* 1976;3:577–588.

Hughes BG, Lawson LD. Antimicrobial effects of *Allium sativum L.* (garlic), *Allium ampeloprasum L.* (elephant garlic), and *Allium cepa L.* (onion), garlic compounds and commercial garlic supplement products. *Phytother Res* 1991;5:154–158.

Ionescu G, et al. Oral citrus seed extract in atopic eczema; in vitro and in vivo studies on intestinal microflora. *J Orthomol Med* 1990;5;3:155–158.

Kamat SA. Clinical trial with berberine hydrochloride for the control of diarrhea in acute gastroenteritis. *J Assoc Physicians India* 1967;15:525–529.

Kaneda Y, et al. In vitro effects of berberine sulfate on the growth of *Entamoeba histolytica, Giardia lamblia,* and *Tricomonas vaginalis. Annals Trop Med Parasitol* 1991;85:417–425.

Kirby GC, O'Neill MJ, Warhurst DC, et al. In vitro studies on the mode of action of quassinoids with activity against chloroquine-resistant *Plasmodium falciparum. Biochem Pharmacol* 1989;38(24):4367–4374.

Krajci WM, Lynch DL. The inhibition of various microorganisms, by crude walnut hulls and juglone. *Microbios Letters* 1997;4:175–181.

Mirelman D, Varon S. Garlic for treatment of Amoebiasis. *Neue Artzliche* 1986;59:10.

Moore GS, Atkins RD. The fungicidal and fungistatic effects of an aqueous garlic extract on medically important yeast-like fungi. *Mycologia* 1997;69:341–348.

Prasad G, Sharma VD. Efficacy of garlic *(Allium sativum)* treatment against experimental candidiasis in chicks. *Br Vet J* 1980;136:448–451.

Rabbani GH, et al. Randomized controlled trial of berberine sulfate therapy for diarrhea due to enterotoxigenic *Escherichia coli* and *Vibrio cholerae. J Infect Dis* 1987;155:979–984.

Sack RB, Froehlich JL. Berberine inhibits intestinal secretory response of *Vibrio cholerae* toxins and *Escherichia coli* enterotoxins. *Infect Immun* 1982;35: 471–475.

Tetsuro I, et al. Isolation and identification of the anti-fungal active substance in walnuts. *Chem Pharm Bull* 1967;15(2):242–245.

Trigg PI. Qinghaosu (artemsinin) as an antimalarial drug. In Wagner J, Hikino H, Farnsworth NR, eds. *Economic and Medicinal Plant Research,* vol. 3. London: Academic Press, 1989.

Tripathi RD, et al. Structure activity relationship amongst some fungitoxic a-naphthoquinones of angiosperm origin. *Agric Biol Chem* 1980;44(10):2483–2485.

Weber ND, et al. In vitro virucidal effects of *Allium sativum* (garlic) extract and compounds. *Plant Medica* 1992;58:417–423.

Xuan-De L, Chia-Chiang S. The chemistry, pharmacology and clinical applications of Qinghaosu *(Artemesinin)* and its derivatives. *Med Res Rev* 1987;7;29–52.

References on Probiotics

Bhatia SJ, Kochar N, Abraham P, Nair NG, Mehta AP. *Lactobacillus acidophilus* inhibits growth of *Campylobacter pylori* in vitro. *J Clin Microbiol* 1989; 27:2328–2330.

Bland, JS. *Applying New Essentials in Nutritional Medicine.* Gig Harbor WA: HealthComm International, 1995.

Chaitow L, Trenev N. *Pro Biotics* London: Thorsons of HarperCollins, 1990.

Clemmesen J. Antitumor effect of *Lactobacillus* substances. "L. bulgaricaus effect." *Mol Biother* 1989;1(15):279–282.

Collins EB, Hardt P. Inhibition of *Candida albicans* by *Lactobacillus acidophilus*. *J Dairy Sci* 1980;5:830–832.

Fernandes CF. Therapeutic role of dietary lactobacilli and lactobacillic fermented dairy products. *FEMS Microbiology Rev* 1987;46:343–356.

Fernandes CF, Shahani KM, Amer MA. Control of diarrhea by lactobacilli. *J Appl Nutr* 1988;40:32–42.

Fernandes CF, Shahani KM. Lactose intolerance and its modulation with *Lactobacilli* and other microbial supplements. *J Appl Nutr* 1989;41;50–64.

Fernandes CF, Shahani KM. Anticarcinogenic and immunological properties of dietary lactobacilli. *J Food Prot* 1990;53:704–710.

Fernandes CF, Shaani KM, Staudinger WL, Amer MA. Mode of tumor suppression by *Lactobacillus acidophilus*. *J Nutr Med* 1991;2:25–34.

Friend BA, Shahani KM. Nutritional and therapeutic aspects of *Lactobacilli*. *J Appl Nutr* 1988;36;2-15;1988

Gilliland SE, et al. Antagonistic action of *Lactobacillus acidophilus* toward intestinal and food-borne pathogens in associative cultures. *J Food Prot* 1977;40:820–823.

Gorbach SL, Chang T, Goldin B. Successful treatment of relapsing *Clostridium difficile* colitis with *Lactobacillus GG*. *Lancet* 1987;26:1519.

Gotz VP, Romankiewics JA, Moss J, Murray HW. Prophylaxis against ampicillin-induced diarrhea with a lactobacillus preparation. *Amer J Hosp Pharm* 1979;36:754–757.

Hamdan IY, Mikolajcik EM. Acidolin: an antibiotic produced by *Lactobacillus acidophilus*. *J Antibiotics* 1974;8;631–636.

Hosono A, et al. Anti-mutagenic properties of lactic acid cultured milk on chemical and fecal mutagens. *J Dairy Sci* 1986;69:2237–2242.

Lidbeck A, Nord CE, Gustafsson JA, Rafter J. Lactobacilli, anticarcinogenic activities and human intestinal microflora. *Eur J Cancer Prev* 1992;1:341–353.

Majamaa H, Isolauri E. Probiotics: a novel approach in the management of food allergy. *J Allergy Clin Immunol* 1997;99:179–185.

Pearce JL, Hamilton JR. Controlled trial or orally administered lactobacilli in acute infantile diarrhea. *J Pediatr* 1974;84:261–262.

Reddy G, et al. Inhibitory effect of yogurt on Ehrlich ascites tumor cell proliferation. *J Natl Cancer Inst* 1973;52:815–817.

Shahani KM, Vakil JR, Kilara A. Natural antibiotic activity of *Lactobacillus acidophilus* and *bulgaricus*. *Cult Dairy Prod J* 1997(2)2:8–11.

Chapter 5

Berg RD. The translocation of normal flora bacteria from the gastrointestinal tract to the mesenteric lymph nodes and other organs. Review. *Microecology Therapy* 1981;11:27–34.

Berg R, Wommack E, Deitch EA. Immunosuppression and intestinal bacterial overgrowth synergistically promote bacterial translocation from the GI tract. *Arch Surg* 1988;123:1359–1364.

Beyer RE. The participation of coenzyme Q in free radical production and anti-oxidation. *Free Rad Biol & Med* 1990;8:545–565.

Bjarnasson I, Williams P, Smethurst P, et al. Intestinal permeability and inflammation in rheumatoid arthritis: effects of non-steroidal anti-inflammatory drugs. *Lancet* 1984;2:1171–1174.

Bjarnason I, Williams P, Smethurst P, et al. Effect of nonsteroidal anti-inflammatory drugs and prostaglandins on the permeability of the human small intestine. *Gut* 1986;27:1292–1297.

Breurer RI, et al. Rectal irrigation with short chain fatty acids for distal ulcerative colitis. *Dig Dis Sci* 1991;36(2):185–187.

Burke A, et al. Nutrition and ulcerative colitis. *Baillieres Clin Gastroenterol* 1997;11(1):153–174.

Busch J, Hammer M, Brunkhorst R, Wagener P. Determination of endotoxin in inflammatory rheumatic diseases—the effect of nonsteroidal anti-inflammatory drugs on intestinal permeability. *J Rheumatol* 1988;47: 156–160.

Crayhon R. *Health Benefits of FOS*, New Canaan, CT: Keats Publishers, 1995.

Deitch EA, et al. The gut as portal of entry for bacteremia: the role of protein malnutrition. *Ann Surg* 1987;205:681–692.

Deitch EA, et al. Bacterial translocation from the gut impairs systemic immunity. *Surgery* 1991;109:269–276.

Falth-Magnusson K, Kjellman N-I, Odelram H, et al. Gastrointestinal permeability in children with cow's milk allergy: effect of milk challenge and sodium cromoglycate assessed with polyethyleneglycols (PEG 400 and PEG 1000). *Clin Allergy* 1984;14:277–286.

Fernandes CF, Shahani KM. Anti-carcinogenic and immunological properties of dietary lactobacilli. *J Food Protection.* 1990;53(8):714–710.

Fishbein L, et al. Fructo-oligosaccharides: a review. *Vet Hum Toxicol* 1988;30(2): 104–107.

Gaby AR. The role of coenzyme Q10 in clinical medicine: part I. *Alterna Med Rev* 1996;1(1):11–17.

Galland L. Leaky gut syndromes: breaking the vicious cycle. *Townsend Letter For Doctors* 1995;145/146:62–68.

Hamilton IH, Cobden I, Rothwell J, Axon ATR. Intestinal permeability in celiac disease: the response to gluten withdrawal and single-dose gluten challenge. *Gut* 1982;23:202–210.

Hemmings WA. The entry of large molecules derived from dietary protein. *Proc Roy Soc Lond* 1978;B 200:175–192.

Hidaka H, et al. Effects of fructo-oligosaccharides on intestinal flora and human health. *Bifidobacteria Microflora* 1986;5(1):37–50.

Hunter JO. Food allergy—or enterometabolic disorder? *Lancet* 1991;338:495–496.

Husby S, Jensenius JC, Svehag SE. Passage of undegraded antigen into the blood of healthy adults. Further characterization of the kinetics of uptake and the size distribution of antigen. *Scand J Immunol* 1986;24:447–455.

Jackson P, et al. Intestinal permeability in patients with eczema and food allergy. *Lancet* 1981;1:1285–1286.

Jass J. Diet, butyric acid and differentiation of gastrointestinal tumors. *Med Hypothesis* 1985;18:113–118.

Jenkins A, Trew DR, Crump BJ, et al. Do non-steroidal anti-inflammatory drugs increase colonic permeability? *Gut* 1991;32:66–69.

Kare MR, Schechter PJ, et al. Direct pathway to the brain. *Science* 1968;163:952–953.

Kohli Y, Suto Y, Kodama T. Effect of hypoxia on acetic acid ulcer of the stomach in rats with or without coenzyme Q10. *Jpn J Exp Med* 1981;51:105–108.

Landi L, Cabrini L, Masotti L, et al. Coenzyme-3 as an anti-oxidant. Its effect on the composition and structural propertyies of phospholipid vesicles. *Cell Biophysics* 1990;16:1–12.

McKellar RC, et al. Metabolism of fructo-oligosaccharides by Bifidobacerium spp. *App Microbiol Biotechnol* 1989;31:537–541.

Nathan D, et al. Increased cell surface EGF receptor expression during butyrate-induced differentiation of human HCT-116 colon tumor cell clones. *Exp Cell Res* 1990;190:76–84.

Okage S, et al. Inhibitory effect of L-glutamine on gastric irritation and back diffusion of gastric acid in response to aspirin in the rat. *Digest Dis* 1975;20:626.

Parrilli G, Iaffaili RV, Capuano G, et al. Changes in intestinal permeability to lactulose induced by cytotoxic chemotherapy. *Cancer Treat Rep* 1982;66:1435–1436.

Planchon P, et al. New stable butyrate derivatives alter proliferation and differentiation in human mammary cells. *Int J Cancer* 1991;48:443–449.

Poillart P, et al. Butyric monosaccharide ester-induced cell differentiation and anti-tumor activity in mice: importance of their prolonged biological effect for clinical application in cancer therapy. *Int J Cancer* 1991;49:89–95.

Prasad K. Butyric acid: a small fatty acid with diverse biological functions. *Life Sciences* 1980;27:1351–1358.

Recker RR. Calcium absorption and achlorhydia. *N Eng J Med* 1985;313 (2):70–73.

Salim AS. Removing oxygen-derived free radicals stimulates healing of ethanol-induced erosive gastritis in the rat. *Digestion* 1990;47:24–28

Salim AS. Oxygen-derived free radicals and the prevention of duodenal ulcer relapse: new approach. *Am J Med Sci* 1990;300:1–6.

Sankaranarayanan K, et al. Effects of sodium butyrate on X-ray and bleomycin induced chromosome aberrations in human peripheral blood lymphocytes. *Gen Res* 1990;56:267–276.

Shive W. Glutamine in treatment of peptic ulcer. *Texas State J Med* 1957;53:.

Souba WW, Klimberg VS, Hautamaki RD, et al. Oral glutamine reduces bacterial translocation following abdominal radiation. *J Surg Res* 1990;48:1–5.

Spaeth G, Berg RD, Specian RD, Deitch EA. Food without fiber promotes bacterial translocation from the gut. *Surgery* 1990;108:240–242.

Steffansson, Dieperink ME, Richman DP, Gomez CM, Marton LS. Sharing of antigenic determinants between the nicotinic acetylcholine receptor and proteins in *Escherichia coli, Proteus vulgaris,* and *Klebsiella pneumoniae.* Possible role in the pathogenesis of *myasthenia gravis. N Engl J Med* 1985;321(4):221–225.

Stoddart J, et al. Sodium butyrate suppresses the transforming activity of an activated N-ras oncogene in human colon carcinoma cells. *Exp Cell Res* 1989;184:16–27.

Tache Y, Wingate D. *Brain-Gut Interactions.* Boca Raton, FL: CRC Press, 1990.

Ukabam SO, Cooper BT. Small intestinal permeability as an indicator of jejunal mucosal recovery in patients with celiac sprue on a gluten-free diet. *J Clin Gastro* 1985;7:232–236.

Well CL, Maddaus MA, Simmons RL. Proposed mechanism for the translocation of intestinal bacteria. *Rev Infect Dis* 1988;10:958–968.

Chapter 6

References on Digestive Enzymes

Dittmar FW, Weissenbacher ER. Therapy of adnexitis—enhancement of the basic antibiotic therapy with hydrolytic enzymes. *Internat J Feto-Maternal Med* 1993;2(3):15–24.

Marsh, et al. Acute pancreatitis following cutaneous exposure to an organophosphate insecticides. *Am J Gastroenterology* 1988;83:1158–1160.

McCarthy CF. Nutritional defects in patients with malabsorption. *Proc Nutr Soc* 1976;35:37–40.

Phelan JJ, et al. Coeliac disease: the abolition of gliadin toxicity by enzymes from *Aspergillus niger. Clin Sci Molec Med* 1977;53:35–43.

Seifert J, et al. Quantitative analysis about the absorption of trypsin, chymotrypsin, amylase, papain, and pancreatin in the GI tract after oral administration. *Gen Physician (Allgemeinarzt),* 1990;19(4):132–137.

References on Lipoic Acid

Bast A, Haenen GRMM. Regulation of lipid peroxidation by glutathione and lipoic acid: involvement of liver microsomal vitamin E free radical reductase. In Emerit I, ed. *Antioxidants in Therapy and Preventive Medicine.* New York: Plenum Press, 1990.

Becker CE, et al. Diagnosis and treatment of amanital phalloides-type mushroom poisoning: use of thioctic acid. *West J Med* 1976;125:100–109.

References

Berkson BM. Alpha-lipoic acid (thioctic acid): my experience with this outstanding therapeutic agent. *J Orthomolec Med* 1998;13(1):48.

Burkart V, Koike T, Brenner HH, et al, Dihydrolipoic acid protects pancreatic islet cells from inflammatory attack. *Agents and actions* 1993;38(1–2):60–65.

Harris JB, et al. Lipoic acid: essential cofactor for gastric secretion. *Fed Proc* 1967;26:273.

Kagan VE, Shveda A, Serbinova E, et al. Dihydrolipoic acid—a universal antioxidant both in the membrane and in the aqueous phase. Reduction of peroxyl, ascorbyl and chromanoxyl radicals. *Biochem Pharmacol* 1992;11(8):1637– 1649.

Marshall E, et al. Treatment of alcohol-related liver disease with thioctic acid: a six month randomised double blind trial. *Gut* 1982;23;1088–1093.

Packer L, Witt EH, Tritschler HJ, et al. Alpha-lipoic acid as a biological antioxidant. *Free Rad Biol Med* 1995;19(2):227–250.

Sen CK, Roy S, Han D, Packer L. Regulation of cellular thiols in human lymphocytes by a-lipoic acid: a flow cytometric analysis. *Free Rad Biol Med* 1997;22(7):1241–1257.

Teutsche C, Brennan RW. Amanita mushroom poisoning with recovery from coma: a case report. *Ann Neurol* 1978;3:177–179.

Other References

Alarcon de la Lastra D, Martin MJ, Motilva V. Antiulcer and gastroprotective effects of quercetin: a gross and histological study. *Pharmacol* 1994;48:56–62.

Bellamy W, et al. Killing of *Candida albicans* by lactoferricin B, a potent antimicrobial peptide derived from the N-terminal region of bovine lactoferrin. *Med Microb Immunol* 1993;182(2):97–205.

Bolla KI, Briefel G, Spector D, et al. Neurocognitive effects of aluminum. *Arch Neurol* 1992;49:1021–1026.

Breneman JC. Allergy elimination diet as the most effective gallbladder diet. *Ann Allergy* 1968;26:83.

Carruthers LB. Chronic diarrhea treated with folic acid. *Lancet* 1946;1:849.

Cheney G. Vitamin U therapy of peptic ulcer. *Calif Med* 1952;77(4):248–252.

Cheney G. Rapid healing of peptic ulcers in patients receiving fresh cabbage juice. *Calif Med* 1949;70:10–14.

Fujita T, Sakurai K. Efficacy of glutamine-enriched enteral nutrition in an experimental model of mucosal ulcerative colitis. *Brit J Surg* 1995;82:749–751.

Forstner GA, et al. Clinical aspects of gastrointestinal mucus. *Adv Exp Med Biol* 1982;144:199–244.

Gledhill T, et al. Epidemic hypochlorhydria. *Br Med J* 1985;289:1383–1386.

Grisham MB. Oxidants and free radicals in inflammatory bowel disease. *Lancet* 1994;344:859–861.

Ellison RT. The effects of lactoferrin on gram-negative bacteria. *Adv Exp Med Biol* 1994;357:371–390.

Hasegawa K. Inhibition with lactoferrin of in vitro infection with human herpes virus. *Jap J Med Sci Biol* 1994;47(2):73–85.

Hornsby-Lewis, Shike M, Brennan MF, et al. L-glutamine supplementation in home total parenteral nutrition patients: stability, safety, and effects on intestinal absorption. *J Parenteral Enteral Nutr* 1994;18(3):268–73.

Iacono G, Cavataio F, Carroccio A, et al. Cow's milk-protein allergy as a cause of anal fistula and fissures: a case report. *J Allergy Clin Immunol* 1998;101(1): 125–127.

Juven B, et al. Studies on the mechanism of the antimicrobial action of oleuropein. *J Appl Bacteriol* 1972;35:559–567.

Kiuchi F, Shiuyu M, Sankawa U. Inhibitors of prostaglandin biosynthesis from ginger. *Chem Pharm Bull* 1982;30:754–757.

Mowrey DB, Clayson DE. Motion sickness, ginger and psychophysics. *Lancet* 1982;1:655–657.

Mossiman BL, White MV, Kaliner MA. Substance P, calcitonin gene-related peptide, and vasoactive intestinal peptide increase in nasal secretions after allergen challenge in atopic patients. *J Allergy Clin Immunol* 1992;1(1):95–105.

O'Connor JB, Richter JE. Recognizing extraesophageal manifestations of GERD. *Intern Med* 1998;19(10):40–48.

Oguchi S, et al. Iron saturation alters the effect of lactoferrin on the proliferation and differentiation of human enterocytes (Caco-2-cells). *Biol Neonate* 1995;67(5):330–339.

Okutomi T, et al. Augmented inhibition of growth of *Candida albicans* by neutrophils in the presence of lactoferrin. *Fems Immunol Med Micro* 1997;18(2):105–112.

Perl DP, Gajdusek DC, Garruto RM, et al. Intraneuronal aluminum accumulation in amyotrophic lateral sclerosis and Parkinsonism-dementia of Guam. *Science* 1982;217:1053–1055.

Rees WRW, Evans BK, Rhodes J. Treating irritable bowel syndrome with peppermint oil. *Brit Med J* 1979; :835.

Rhodes JM, Parker N, Ching CK, Patel P. Mucin subclasses in ulcerative colitis. *Gastroenterology* 1987;93(2):435–436.

Samaranayaki YH. The antifungal effect of lactoferrin and lysozyme on *Candida krusei* and *Candida albicans*. *Apmis* 1997;105(11):875–883.

Satoskar RR, Shah SJ, Shenoy SG. Evaluation of anti-inflammatory property of curcumin (diferuloyl methane) in patients with postoperative inflammation. *Internat J Clin Pharmacol Ther Toxicol* 1986:24:651–654.

Shimmura S, et al. Subthreshhold UV radiation-induced peroxide formation in cultured corneal epithelial cells: the protective effects of lactoferrin. *Exp Eye Res* 1996;63(5):519–526.

Shive W, et al. Glutamine in treatment of peptic ulcer. *Texas State J Med* 1957.

Somerville K, et al. Delayed release peppermint oil capsules (Colpermin) for the spastic colon syndrome: a pharmacokinetic study. *Brit J Clin Pharmacol* 1984;18:638–640.

Thornton JR, Emmett PM, Heaton KW. Diet and gallstones: effects of refined carbohydrate diets on bile cholesterol saturation and bile acid metabolism. *Gut* 1983;24:2.

Tranter HS, Tassou SC, Nychas GJ. The effect of the olive phenolic compound, oleuropein, on growth and enterotoxin B production by *Staphylococcus aureus*. *J Appl Bacteriol* 1993;74:253–259.

Trauner M, Meier PJ, Boyer JL. Molecular pathogenesis of cholestasis. *New Engl J Med* 1998;339(17):1217–1227.

Walker M. *Olive Leaf Extract*. New York: Kensington Books, 1997.

Weberg R, Rerstad A. Gastrointestinal absorption of aluminum from single doses of aluminum-containing antacids in man. *Eur J Clin Invest* 1986;16:428–432.

Werbach MR. *Nutritional Influences on Illness*. New Canaan, CT: Keats Publishers, 1988.

Ziegler TR, Benfell K, Wilmore DW, et al. Safety and metabolic effects of L-glutamine administration in humans. *J Paren Enter Nutr* 1990;14(4 Suppl): 137S–146S.

Chapter 7

Anonymous. New misgivings about magnesium. *Science News* 1988;133(32):356.

Bernard EM, Wong B, Armstrong D. Sterioisomeric configuration of arabinitol in serum, urine, and tissues in invasive candidiasis. *J Infect Dis* 1985;151(4): 711–715.

Brandtzeg P. Research in gastrointestinal immunology state of the art. *Scand J Gastroenterol* 1985;114:137–156.

Cattaneo M, et al. High prevalence of hyperhomocysteinemia in patients with inflammatory bowel disease: a pathogenic link with thromboembolie complications? *Thromb Haemost* 1998;80:543–545.

Clapp S. Case control studies for Campylobacter to begin in October. *Food & Chem News* 1997;39(27):7.

Das UN. Hypothesis: cis-unsaturated fatty acids as potential anti-peptic ulcer drugs. *Prost-glandins, Leukot Essent Fatty Acids* 1998;58(5):377–380.

Gittleman AL. *Guess What Came To Dinner*. Garden City, NJ: Avery Publishers, 1993.

Iacono G, Cavataio F, Carroccio A, et al. Intolerance to cow's milk and chronic constipation in children. *New Eng J Med* 1998;339:1100–1104.

Iacono G, et al. Cow's milk-protein allergy as a cause of anal fistula and fissures: a case report. *New Engl J Med* 1998;101;1(1):125–127.

Lagergren J, Bergstrom R, Lingren A, Nyren O. Symptomatic gastroesophageal reflux as a risk factor for esophageal adenocarcinoma. *New Eng J Med* 1999;340:825–831.

Marier JR. Magnesium content of the food supply in the modern-day world. *Magnesium* 1986;5:1–8.

Mosimann BL, White MV, Kaliner MA, et al. Substance P, calcitonin gene-related peptide, and vasoactive intestinal peptide increase in nasal secretions after allergen challenge in atopic patients. *J Allergy Clin Immunol* 1993;92:95–104.

Present DH, Rutgerts P, van Deventer SJH. Infliximab for the treatment of fistulas in patients with Crohn's disease. *New Engl J Med* 1999;340:14398–14405.

Roboz J. Diagnosis and monitoring of disseminated candidiasis based on serum/urine D/L-arabinitol ratios. *Chirality* 1994:6(2):51–57.

Rose JB. Environmental ecology of Cryptosporidium and public health implications. *Ann Rev Public Health* 1997;18:135–161.

Schroeder HA. Losses of vitamins and trace minerals resulting from processing and preservation of foods. *Am J Clin Nutr* 1971;24;564–573.

Seelig MS. Nutritional status and requirements of magnesium. *Mag Bull* 1986;8:170–185.

Sell D, Monnier V. Structure elucidation of a senescence cross-link from human extracellular matrix. Implication of pentoses in the aging process. *J Biol Chem* 1989; 264:21597–21602.

Stenson WF, Cort D, Becken W, et al. Dietary supplementation with fish oil in ulcerative colitis. *Ann Int Med* 1992;116:609–614.

Stotland BR, Cirigliano MD, Lichtenstein GR. Medical therapies for inflammatory bowel disease. *Hospital Practice* 1998; :141–168.

Tamm. Biochemical activity of intestinal microflora in adult coeliac disease. *Nahrung* 1984;28:711–715.

Van der Heiden C. Gas chromatographic analysis of urinary tryosine and phenylalanine metabolites in patients with gastrointestinal disorders. *Clinical Chimia Acta* 1971;345:289–296.

Vojdani A, Rahimian P, Kalhor H, Mordechai E. Immunological cross reactivity between *Candida albicans* and human tissue. *J Clin Lab Immunol* 1996;48: 1–15.

Whang R, Qu TO, Aikowa JK, et al. Predictors of clinical hypomagnesemia and hypermagnesemia, requested versus routine. *J Amer Med Assoc* 1990; 263: 3036–3064.

Note: Each laboratory listed has voluminous references on their tests available to physicians.

Resource Guide

I'll bet you were wondering where you could find the healing remedies discussed throughout this book. This section has it all: mail order sources for products, laboratories for tests, organizations to contact for finding a doctor, lists of companies and their products, as well as a list of recommended books for more information.

Note: asterisks (*) refer to companies whose products come highly recommended by people I respect.

Sources for Non-Prescription Supplements

N.E.E.D.S. 1-800-634-1380
527 Charles Ave., 12-A
Syracuse NY 13209
(N.E.E.D.S. has carried everything I prescribe for over a decade, even difficult to find items and items normally only available through nutritionally-trained physicians or in bulk order.)

Wellness Pharmacy 1-800-227-2627
College Pharmacy 1-800-888-9358
Apothecure 1-800-969-6601
Abrams Royal Pharmacy 1-800-458-0804
American Environmental
Health Foundation 1-800-428-2343
Emerson Ecologics 1-800-240-9912/ 654-4432
NutriSupplies 1-800-388-8808
Metagenics 1-800-647-6100

Plus all major nutritional supplement lines.

Sources for Prescription Leaky Gut Test Solution, Nystatin Pure Powder for Candida, etc.

Wellness Pharmacy 1-800-227-2627
College Pharmacy 1-800-888-9358
Apothecure 1-800-969-6601
Abrams Royal Pharmacy 1-800-458-0804
Source of Nystatin Pure Powder (Bio-Statin) for Candida:
Bio-Tech 1-800-345-1199

Tests (Can Only Be Ordered By A Physician):

Note: The labs listed below have many more tests than I have mentioned
that might also be of interest to readers.

Great Smokies Diagnostic Laboratory 1-800-455-4762; (704) 253-1127
63 Zillicoa St.
Asheville NC 28801-1074

Tests:
7 Day Candida test
CDSA (comprehensive stool and digestive analysis)
Purged parasites
Leaky gut test (intestinal permeability)
Quantitative H. pylori antibodies
Vitamin panel
Mineral and heavy metal panel
Fatty acid analysis
Candida antibodies
Food allergy antibodies
Amino acid

MetaMetrix Laboratory 1-800-221-4640; (770) 441-2237
5000 Peachtree Ind. Blvd, Suite 110
Norcross GA 30071

Tests:
Mineral panel or Elemental Analysis on Erythrocytes
Heavy metal panel
Fatty acid panel
Candida Antibodies

Organic Acids
IgG4 & IgE Food Antibody Assays
Amino acids
SMAC
Candida antibodies

Doctor's Data 1-800-323-2784 or 630-231-9190
P.O.Box 111
West Chicago IL 60185

Tests:
W hole blood elements (minerals and heavy metals)
Amino acids
Fecal toxic elements

ImmunoSciences Lab, Inc. 1-800-950-4686; (310) 657-1053
8730 Wilshire Blvd., Suite 305
Beverly Hills, CA 90211

Tests:
Specialty tests for H pylori antibodies, Candida antibodies and sensitivity to environmental chemicals, cancer vulnerability as well as hidden metastases.

American Environmental Health Foundation
1-800-428-2343
8345 Walnut Hill Lane
Dallas TX, 75231

Tests your daily drinking water. Does not require physician prescription. Call for price and information about sending a sample of your water for analysis for undesirable contaminants that hold back health.

Where can I find a doctor who does this kind of medicine?

I am asked this question constantly. Two organizations comprised of physicians who are geared more toward cause and cure medicine versus drug-driven medicine are listed below. It does not mean that every physician in each organization does all of the things you have learned here; some do more, some do less.

American Academy of Environmental Medicine
7701 E Kellogg ST.
Wichita KS 67207
Phone: 316-683-2236
E-mail: *aaem@aol.com*

American College for Advancement in Medicine
23121 Verdugo Dr., Ste 204
Laguna Hills CA 92653
Phone: 949-583-7666
Fax: 949-455-9679
Web site: www.acam.org

If you prefer a list of physicians in your area who have actually taken and passed the board examinations for environmental medicine, send a self-addressed, stamped envelope to the following organization:

American Board of Environmental Medicine
65 Wehrle Dr.
Buffalo NY 14225

Manufacturers of Quality Nutrients Referred to In This Book

The products listed below are available through mail order companies (see the list at the start of this resource section), health food stores and health professionals. To find out where to obtain these products, you can contact the manufacturers directly.

Proper Nutrition, Inc.
1-800-555-8868
web site: www.propernutrition.com

Intestive™

This all-natural dietary supplement offers total gastrointestinal support to sufferers of IBS (Irritable Bowel Syndrome), ulcerative colitis, Crohn's, and those with general intestinal and bowel complaints. Reports and recent re-search indicate that Intestive™ is effective in reducing symptoms related to IBS, including diarrhea, and constipation, and in correcting leaky gut. The predominant ingredient in Intestive is Seacure®, which was previously mentioned in this book as an important source of predigested protein that nourishes a damaged gut. Intestive is a new and improved product that provides Seacure enhanced with the benefits of colostrum (free of lactose and casein) and boswellia, an anti-inflammatory botanical. Take two to four capsules, two to three times a day before meals. Seacure is a whole food concentrate from white fish that provides high quality protein in the form of bioactive peptides and biogenic amines; omega-3 fatty acids; and minerals, phospholipids, and other valuable nutrients present in fish. Dietary peptides are protein fractions that have action in the body beyond their nutritive value as a protein.

The process used to produce Seacure was developed 40 years ago under the aegis of the U.S. National Academy of Sciences in an effort to transform underutilized fish into a supplement to combat world malnutrition. Comprehensive testing confirmed the product's safety and no presence of side effects. Clinical trials and use by health care practitioners later identified Seacure's effectiveness in intestinal healing. Proper Nutrition is a company that has been eager to show me their quality analyses from independent laboratories and supply me with scientific references to back their products. These are important criteria that I look for before I will trust a company with my patients' welfare. Ordering and a wealth of information are available at their web site or order by phone, and all Proper Nutrition products are also available through N.E.E.D.S.

Tyler Encapsulations
2204-8 NW Birdsdale
Gresham, OR 97030
1-800-869-9705

Tyler's products are available through mail order or through health professionals. They also have a line called Prevail whose products are available in health food stores (see the listing following this one).

Multiplex-1 without iron
Paragard
Eskimo-3
Fiber Formula
Candida Complex
Enterogenic Concentrate
Permeability Factors
Similase

Fiber Formula
Detoxification Factors
OxyPerm
PanPlex 2-Phase
Recancostat
Buffered C Powder
Cyto-Redoxin
Betaine HCL
Butyrate enema

Prevail
2204-8 Birdsdale
Gresham, OR 97030
1-800-248-0885
E-mail: *info@prevail.com*

Prevail's products are available through health food stores. Contact Prevail directly for product information and for the store nearest you.

Advance Multi-Vitamin with Enzymes:
Similar to Tyler's Multiplex-1 without iron.

Paragard Relief :
Comparable to Tyler's Paragard.

Eskimo-3:
Identical to Tyler's Eskimo-3.

Inner Ecology :
Comparable to Tyler's Enterogenic Concentrate. Contains FOS, probiotics of Lactobacillus and Bifidus species plus cellulase. Take 1-2 teaspoons in 8 ounces of water between meals, 1-2 times a day.

Vitase Digestive Formula:
Comparable to Tyler's Similase. Contains protease, amylase, lipase, cellulase, lactase, sucrase and maltase. Take 1-2 at the start of meals.

Acid-Ease:
For heartburn and indigestion. Contains the same enzymes as above plus gamma oryzanol, slippery elm and marshmallow root. Take 1-2 at the start of meals.

Detox Enzyme Formula:
Comparable to Tyler's Detoxification Factors. Contains enzymes, antioxidants, amino acids, minerals and vitamins, plus glutathione, N-acetylcysteine, carnitine, calcium D-Glucarate and other minerals that support detoxification. Take 1-2 between meals, 1-2 times a day.

Fat Enzyme Formula:
For difficulty in digesting fats. Contains enzymes with emphasis on lipase. Take 1-2 at the start of meals.

Fiber Enzyme Formula:
For difficulty in digesting fiber. Contains enzymes with emphasis on cellulase. Take 1-2 at the start of meals.

Bean and Vegi Enzyme Formula:
For difficulty in digesting beans, legumes and cruciferous vegetables. Contains enzymes with an emphasis on galactosidase. Take 1-2 at the start of meals.

Children's Digestive Formula:
Multiple digestive enzymes for children aged 3-14. Take 1-2 at the start of meals.

Multi-Vitamin and Minerals:
Contains multiple digestive enzymes coupled with a daily vitamin-mineral preparation. Take 1-2 caps, 2-3 times a day.
Metabolic Liver Formula:
Contains enzymes, silymarin, bile, liver, iodine from kelp, and other liver support nutrients. Take 1-2 caps, 1-3 times a day with meals.

GSH Cell Support:
Contains glutathione, l-cysteine and anthocyanidins to recycle GSH. Take 1-4 between meals, 1-3 times a day.
Antioxidants:
Contains enzymes, key vitamins, minerals, and plant extracts proven through voluminous research to be potent antioxidants like procyanidins, silymarin, glucosinolates, lycopenes, allicin, catechins, and more. Take 1-2 caps, 1-3 times a day with meals.

Defense Formula:
Contains enzymes, thymus, Echinacea, Astragalus, Ligustrum, Shiitake, St. John's Wort, and other boosters for infection fighting. Take one cap, 2-3 times a day.

Klaire Laboratories
1-800-533-7255
1573 W. Seminole
San Marcos CA 92069-2589
Email: *sara@klaire.com*

(10% discount if you mention this book)

Vital Plex
Aloe Vera Drink
Vital-Dophilus
Vital Immune Biotic
Fiber-Plex
Pancreas
Ultra Fine Ascorbic Acid Powder

HealthComm International, Inc.
1-800-843-9660
P.O. Box 1729
5800 Soundview Dr.
Gig Harbor WA 98335

(Available through mail order companies—see list at start of resource section)

UltraClear
Ultra Fiber
UltraInflamX

Enzymatic Therapy
1-800-553-2370/ 1-800-376-7889
825 Challenger Dr
Green Bay WI 54311

(Available in health food stores)

Garlinase
ZymeDophilus
Fiber Plus
Candimyacin
Rhizinate (DGL)

Gastro-Relief (DGL with antacid)
GingerMax
Laxatol
Bromelain Complex
Bio-Zyme

Pure Body Institute
1-800-952-PURE

(10% discount if you mention this book)Nature's Cleansing Program
Pure Body Program

Metabolic Maintenance
1-800-772-7873
68994 North Pine St.
Box 3600
Sister OR 97759

Lipoic Acid 300mg

Pure Encapsulations
1-800-753-2277
5-490 Boston Post Rd.
Sudbury MA 01776
www.pureencapsulations.com

L-Carnitine
A.C. Formula
Lactobacillus sporogenes
Garlic 100:1
Nutra Flax 1000
DGL Plus

Carlson Laboratories
1-800-323-4141
15 College Dr.
Arlington Heights IL 60004-1985

(Available in health food stores)

Cod Liver Oil
Vitamin B6 Liquid
HCl and Pepsin
Cardi-Rite
Mild-C Crystals
ACES Gold
Aloe Gel Caps
E-Gems 800

Thorne
1-800-228-1966
P.O.Box 3200
Sandpoint ID 83864
E-mail: *Info@thorne.com*

Manganese picolinate
Black Current Oil
Citricidin
L. sporogenes
Herbal Bulk
Undecyn
Whey
Formula SF734
L-Glutamine
Biogest
Herbal Laxative
Betaine HCl
Dipan-9
M.F. Bromelain
Basic Nutrients II
Pure Ascorbic Acid Powder
Magnesium Aspartate
Magnesium Citrate
Plant Antioxidants
Super EPA
Phytosome

American Lecithin Co.
1-800-364-4416
115 Hurley Rd., Unit 2B
Oxford CT 06478

Phos Chol Concentrate

Longevity Science/ Klabin Marketing
1-800-933-9440
2067 Broadway, Suite 700
N.Y., NY 10023

BioPro-A Thymic
MSM

Nutricology
1-800-545-9960/ 1-800-782-4274
30806 Santana St
P.O.Box 55907
Hayward CA 94544

ParaMicrocidin
Oil of Oregano
Organic Pancreas
Magnesium 18% Solution
BottomsUp
L-Glutamine Powder
Artemesia 500 mg
MSM
Laktoferrin
Butyren

Ecologic Formulas/ Cardiovascular Research
1-800-888-4585
1061-B Shary Circle
Concord, CA 94518

Cal-Mag Butyrate
Nutricillin
Sialex

Chromium Cruciferate
Soy-Free Phosphatides
Allithiamine
Kapricidin-A
Paracan-Myc
Laktoferrin
Helicobactrin
Gastro Met

Wakunaga of America
1-800-825-7888/ 1-800-421-2998
23501 Madero
Mission Viejo CA 92691

(Available in health food stores. You can get free samples if you mention
this book.)

Kyodophilus
Kyolic
Kyo-Green
Whey

Jarrow
1-800-726-0886/ 1-800-890-8955
1824 S. Robertson Blvd
Los Angeles CA 90035-4317

(Available in health food stores)

L-Carnitine
Jarrow-Dophilus
Flax Fiber
Yaemama Chlorella
Whey
L-Glutamine
Bromelain
L-Arginine
Magnesium citrate + K + Taurine
MSM

T.A.D. Corp
1-800-326-0256
560 River Road, Fair Haven NJ 07704

AquaPhase A

Bio-Botanical Research, Inc.
408-724-4140
P.O.Box 1061
Soquel CA 95073

Biocidin

American Biologics
1-800-227-4473
1180 Walnut Ave
Chula Vista CA, 91911

Dioxychlor DC3

Natren
1-800-992-3323
Many varieties of probiotics

UAS Laboratories
800-422-3371
5610 Rowland Rd. #110
Minnetonka MN 55343
Many varieties of probiotics

Aloe Products of N. America
315-492-8372
Syracuse NY, 13205

(10% discount if you mention this book)

Aloe Vera Drink

WaterOz
800-547-2294
P.O. Box 159
Stites ID 83552-1259

Silver Mineral Water

BioTech
1-800-345-1199
Box 1992
Fayetteville AR 72702

(10% discount if you mention this book)

Bromase
Digest III
Glutamine
Bio-Statin (Nystatin Rx)
PCN-200
L-Glutathione

Neesby
1-800-633-7294

Mycopryl

Emerson Ecologics
1-800-240-9912/ 1-800-654-4432

Efamol's Evening Primrose Oil

Environmental Health Link
419-659-5541

Stevia

Scientific Consultant
1-800-632-2370

Tanalbit

Phillips Nutritionals
1-800-514-5115
27071 Cabot Rd, Ste 122
Laguna Hills CA 92653

Bromelain
Evening Primrose Oil
Garlic Supreme
OptiQ-100

Carotec, Inc.
1-800-522-4279
P.O. Box 9919
Naples, FL 34101

Ulva Rigida (glucuronic acid)
Wobenzyme enzymes

Solgar Vitamin & Herb
1-800-645-2246
500 Willow Tree Road
Leonia, NJ 07605

(Available in health food stores)

Acidophilus
Acidophilus Plus
Bromelain 500
Digestive Aide
Organic Garlic 500
Evening Primrose Oil 500
Flax Seed Oil
L-Glutamine
Psyllium Husks Fiber 500

Source Naturals
1-800-815-2333
23 Janis Way
Scotts Valley, CA 96066

(Available in health food stores)

Super Carrot Acidophilus
Activated Quercetin
Bromelain
Citricidex
Grapefruit Pectin
Ultra-Mag
Life Flora
Ultra Colloidal Silver

Products For A Cleaner Environment

E.L.Foust
1-800-EL-FOUST/ 1-800-353-6878
P.O. Box 105
Elmhurst IL 60126

Air purifiers for home, office, and car

American Environmental Health Foundation
1-800-428-2343
8345 Walnut Hill Lane
Dallas TX, 75231

Test your daily drinking water. Call for price and information about sending a sample of your water for analysis for undesirable contaminants that hold back health. Also water filters, air filters, health books, cleaning products, cotton products and many other catalog items for healthier home environment.

N.E.E.D.S.
(800) 634-1380

Carries a full line of air and water filters and products that contribute toward detoxification.

Nontoxic Environments, Inc.
1-800-789-4348
P.O. Box 384
Newmarket NH 03867
www.nontoxicenvironments.com

Water filters, cleaning products and other products for a healthier home.

Janice Corp
1-800-JANICES
198 Rte 46
Budd Lake NJ 07828
Website: *www.janice.com*

Cotton bedding, mattresses and some clothes

Mountain Green™
1-888-878-5781
7399 South Tucson Way
Englewood, CO 80112
www.mtngreen.com

Manufacturers of environmentally responsible household cleaning products that are biodegradable and non-toxic. They do not contain harsh chemicals such as EDTA, NTA, chlorine bleach, dyes, perfumes, phosphates, or optical brighteners.

Ultra Liquid and Ultra Powdered Laundry Detergents, Fabric Softener, Natural Orange and Natural Apple Dishwashing Liquids, Glass Cleaner Spray, and other cleaning products.

Harmony
1-800-869-3446
360 Interlocken Blvd., Suite 300
Broomfield, CO 80004

Air purifiers for the home and to wear on the body, full spectrum lights, water filters, cleaning products, cotton bedding and clothes.

*Allens Naturally®
1-800-352-8971
P.O. Box 514
Farmington, MI 48332-0514
www.allensnaturally.com

Manufacturer of biodegradable and non-toxic household cleaning products that are free of perfumes and dyes and don't involve any animal testing or animal-based ingredients.

Biodegradable Heavy Duty All Purpose Cleaner, Biodegradable Fruit and Veggie Wash, Liquid Laundry Detergent, Biodegradable Anti Static Fabric Softener, Non Toxic Glass and Surface Cleaner, and other cleaning products. This line of cleansers is also available through N.E.E.D.S.

Product for Detoxification

Far Infrared Therapy Sauna

High Tech Health
1-800-794-5355
www.hightechhealth.com

Thermal Life® Far Infrared Therapy Sauna
    This highly effective low-temperature sauna (100F to 130F) employs heaters that emit rays at a special wavelength designed to push heavy metal toxins, including mercury and other toxins, out of the body. There have been reports of high mercury levels coming down substantially—some cases have become mercury-free in 90 days. More than 500 doctors in the U.S. are now providing this therapy for their patients. The best part of this sauna is its ease of use. It requires no pre-heating, doesn't need any water,

and it can be moved anywhere in the home or apartment. Unit sizes available for 1-5 persons. This sauna is constructed using poplar wood so there will be no out-gassing of terpines that will contribute to total toxicity.

Natural Cosmetics

Carlson
1-800-323-4141

E Gem Shampoo with Natural Vitamin E, E Gem Glycerine Soap with Vitamins E and A and no animal ingredients, ADE(Intensive Moiturizing Cream with Natural Vitamin E, Key˙E® Moisturizing Cream with Natural Vitamin E, Key˙E® Soothing Ointment with Natural Vitamin E, and many others.

Jason Natural Cosmetics
1-800-JASON-05
www.jason-natural.com

Chamomile Liquid Satin Soap™ with Pump
Natural Sea Kelp Shampoo

Jason Natural carries a full line of cosmetics that are free of toxic substances, including natural underarm deodorant and alcohol-free shaving cream and after-shave lotion.

*The Natural Place, Inc.
1-914-352-7331

Manufacturer of Superlan® cream for dry, chapped lips (in a convenient flow-on applicator) and Superlan® Lite moisturizer for dry skin. Both products are made with only hypo-allergenic lanolin and organic jojoba oil and no pesticides or impurities.

Suppliers of Organic and Whole Food Products

Lundberg Family Farms
1-530-882-4550 (ext. 319)
5370 Church Street
P.O. Box 369
Richvale, CA 95974-0369
www.lundberg.com

Grower and marketer of organic rice and rice products, including short, medium and long grain, sweet rice, Wehani, Black Japonica, California basmati, jasmine and arborio, and other varieties. They also carry organic brown rice pasta. Available in health food stores.

*Amy's Kitchen
1-707-578-7188
P.O. Box 449
Petaluma, CA 94953

Makers of natural and organic frozen meals, canned soups and bottled pasta sauces that are sold in natural food stores, groceries and supermarkets.

Capilano Pacific
1-877-391-WILD (9453)
www.capilanopacific.com

Wildfish™
This company is a wonderful source for wild-caught salmon. Most of the salmon available in restaurants and stores are farm-raised. Usually this means medications such as antibiotics have been added to the feed, as well as synthetic coloring. Wild-caught salmon has none of these problems and a high level of omega-3 fatty acids and much less fat than farm-raised salmon. It tastes better as well. Also available: halibut, tuna and lox without any added chemicals.

*Crown Prince
1-800-255-5063
18581 Railroad Street
City of Industry, CA 91748

Canned fish (caught in the wild) including Brisling sardines packed in olive oil or water, pink salmon and albacore tuna.

Sheltons Poultry, Inc.
1-800-541-1844
204 Loranne Ave.
Pomona, CA 91767-5798

Free-range and antibiotic-free chickens and turkeys, available in natural foods stores.

Spectrum Naturals
1-800-995-2705
133 Copeland Street
Petaluma, CA 94952

Spectrum Naturals carries a full line of oils, including unrefined extra virgin olive oil and organic flax oils. Spectrum Organic Products offers a wide range of organic foods, including Millina's Healthy Kitchen organic pastas and pasta sauces with added omega-3 fatty acids for heart health.

Whole Foods Catalogues

Even if you don't live near a big city or health food store, you can get tea tree oil, stevia, quality organic whole grains and beans, nuts and other foods from these sources by mail:

Natural Lifestyle   1-800-752-2775
16 Outlook Dr
Asheville NC 28804-3330

Omega Nutrition USA   1-800-661-3529
6515 Aldrich Road
Bellingham, WA 98226
www.omeganutrition.com

Kushi Institute Store   1-800-645-8744
P.O. Box 500
Becket, MA 01223-0500

Recommended Books for More Information

By Dr. William Crook: 1-800-227-2627
The Yeast Connection
The Yeast Connection Cookbook

By Dr. John Parks Trowbridge and Dr. Morton Walker: 1-800-223-6834
The Yeast Syndrome

Books and Services by Sherry A. Rogers, M.D.

Total Wellness™—This referenced monthly newsletter will keep you up to date on new findings. In this era, because we cannot get the information out to you fast enough, we use the newsletter as our communication link. It will teach you useful facts years before they will be presented elsewhere, and it is practical and action-oriented. Just as important as the new is the integration of the new with what you have already learned. For if you lack explicit directions on how to implement it in your life, what good is it? For mere pennies a day, you really cannot afford to be without the most practical resource of all. (12 Issues per year)

Wellness Against All Odds—Here is the 6th and most revolutionary book by Sherry A. Rogers, M.D. It contains the ultimate healing plan that people have successfully used to beat cancer when they were given 2 weeks, some even 2 days to live by some of the top medical centers. These people had exhausted all that medicine has to offer, including surgery, chemotherapy, radiation and bone marrow transplants. And one of the most unbelievable things is that the plan costs practically nothing to implement and most of it can be done at home with non-prescription items. Of course, in keeping with the other works and going far beyond, this contains the mechanisms of how these principles heal and is complete with all the scientific references for physicians.

Depression Cured at Last!— Are you depressed, blue, down in the dumps? Do you lack a reason for being, lack motivation, lack a zest for life, lack zip? Do you feel you need a jump start, need to be ignited with a passion that will fuel you with excitement? Is it difficult to awaken feeling happy, healthy and full of enthusiasm for the new day? Wouldn't you like to learn how to turn on the "happy hormones" in your brain? You now can possess the tools with which to find the causes and cures.

The E.I. Syndrome, Revised—This book is 650 pages crammed full of pearls and spells out the entire work-up for the most mildly allergic person to the universal reactor, which Dr. Rogers, herself was. It goes through everything the patient needs to know about mold and other inhalant allergies, food allergies, chemical allergies, Candida syndrome, nutritional deficiencies, toxicities of xenobiotics, and the psychoneuroimmune connection. It shows you how to diagnose your own food and mold allergies and chemical sensitivities. Then it tells you how to treat them, with environmental controls and diet changes you can do at home. This is required reading for all people with environmental illness, regardless of the stage.

You Are What You Ate—This book is macrobiotics modified for the chemically sensitive person and people with mysterious undiagnosable illnesses as well as those who have been told they just have to learn to live with it. It is for people who have severe cravings, resistant Candidiasis, or who have had food injections, rotation diets, vitamins and everything they can think of, but are still not functioning at 100%. This is required reading before tackling the more advanced stage in "The Cure Is In The Kitchen."

The Cure Is In The Kitchen—Did you ever read the books about people who cleared their cancers with macrobiotics and find yourself asking "Well, what did they eat and do day to day?" Dr. Rogers did and went straight to the highest source to find the answer. This is the first book to ever spell out in detail what all those people ate day to day who cleared their incurable diseases, undiagnosable symptoms, relentless chemical, food, Candida and electromagnetic sensitivities, as well as terminal cancers. Dr. Rogers flew to Boston each month to work side by side with Michio Kushi as he counseled people at the end of their medical ropes, as their remarkable case histories will show you.

Macro Mellow—This book is designed for 4 types of people:
    (1) For the person who doesn't know a thing about macrobiotics, but just plain wants to feel better, in spite of the 21st century.
    (2) It solves the high cholesterol/triglycerides problem without drugs and is the perfect diet for heart disease patients.
    (3) It is the perfect transition diet for those not ready for macro, but needing to get out of the chronic illness rut.
    (4) It spells out how to feed the rest of the family who hates macro while another family member must eat it to clear their incurable symptoms. The delicious low-fat whole food meals use macro ingredients without the rest of the family even knowing. It is the first book to dove-tail creative meal planning, menus, recipes and even gardening so that it doesn't drive the cook (who used to have to run 2 kitchens, "normal" & strict macro) crazy!

Tired or Toxic?—Here is the first book, complete with references that provides in terms that everyone can understand, the biochemical explanation and verification of chemical hypersensitivity, Candida sensitivity, and how to heal all of these, including some cancers. It explains the most common biochemical blunders of medicine, and how they actually promote aging, Alzheimer's and arteriosclerosis. These blunders include the prescription drugs to lower cholesterol, the prescription of blood pressure medication, the recommendation of calcium for osteoporosis, and drugs for arthritis. Medicine is on the threshold of another stage in its evolution. No longer is a headache a Darvon deficiency. We now have the tools to identify and correct the environmental triggers and nutritional and biochemical deficiencies that cause disease, rather than just drugging or covering up symptoms. If you want to bring your doctor into the 21st century, this is the book to give him.

Chemical Sensitivity—This 48 page booklet is the most concise referenced booklet on chemical sensitivity. It is for the person wanting to learn about it but who is leery of tackling a big book. It is ideal for teaching your physician or convincing your insurance company, as it is fully referenced. It is a good reference for the veteran who wants a quick concise review. If you are not completely well, you need to read this book. If you have been sentenced to a life-time of drugs, whether it be for high blood pressure, high cholesterol, angina, arrhythmia, asthma, eczema, sinusitis, colitis, learning disabilities, or cancer, you need this book. It matters not what your label is. What matters is whether chemical sensitivity is a factor that no one has explored that is keeping you from getting well. Most probably it is, and this is an inexpensive way to find out.

The Scientific Basis for Selected Environmental Medicine Techniques— This book contains the scientific evidence and references for many of the techniques of environmental medicine. It is designed for patients who choose to find the causes of their illnesses rather than merely mask their symptoms with drugs for the rest of their lives. It is also for those who have been unfairly denied insurance coverage. It is the ideal book with which to educate your PTA, attorney, insurance company, or physicians who still doubt your sanity, or who doubt that environmental medicine lacks scientific back-up.

Phone consultations—Many people are stuck. They have an undiagnosable condition. Or they have a label but have been unable to get well. Or they have a "dead-end" label which means nothing more can be done. And many are not able to find a physician who is trained in what our 9 books explore. These people could benefit from a personal consultation with Dr. Sherry Rogers to explore what diagnostic and treatment options may exist that they or their physicians are not aware of. For this reason we offer prepaid, scheduled phone consultations with the doctor. These can be scheduled through the office by calling (315) 488-2856.

Price List:
Total Wellness™ $39.95
Wellness Against All Odds $17.95
Depression Cured At Last! $24.95
E.I. Syndrome $17.95
You Are What You Ate $12.95
The Cure is in the Kitchen $14.95
Macro Mellow $12.95
Tired or Toxic? $18.95
Chemical Sensitivity $3.95
Scientific Basis for Selected Env. Med. Techniques $17.95

Shipping/handling on book orders only: $4.00 for first item with $1.00 for each additional item.

Prestige Publishing, PO Box 3068, Syracuse, NY 13220
1-800-846-6687 ♦315-455-7862 ♦Fax 315-454-8119
Email: orders@prestigepublishing.com

Metric Conversion Charts

Formulas for conversion

Fahrenheit to Celsius: subtract 32, multiply by 5, then divide by 9
for example:

$$212°F - 32 = 180$$
$$180 \times 5 = 900$$
$$900 \div 9 = 100°C$$

Celsius to Fahrenheit: multiply by 9, the divide by 5, then add 32
for example:

$$100°C \times 9 = 900$$
$$900 \div 5 = 180$$
$$180 + 32 = 212°F$$

Temperatures (Fahrenheit to Celsius)

−10°F =	−23°C	coldest part of freezer
0°F =	−17°C	freezer
32°F =	0°C	water freezes
68°F =	20°C	room temperature
85°F =	29°C	
100°F =	38°C	
115°F =	46°C	water simmers
135°F =	57°C	water scalds
140°F =	60°C	
150°F =	66°C	

Temperatures (Fahrenheit to Celsius)

160°F = 71°C
170°F = 77°C
180°F = 82°C   water simmers
190°F = 88°C
200°F = 95°C
205°F = 96°C   water simmers
212°F = 100°C   water boils, at sea level
225°F = 110°C
250°F = 120°C   very low (or slow) oven
275°F = 135°C   very low (or slow) oven
300°F = 150°C   low (or slow) oven
325°F = 165°C   low (or moderately slow) oven
350°F = 180°C   moderate oven
375°F = 190°C   moderate (or moderately hot) oven
400°F = 205°C   hot oven
425°F = 220°C   hot oven
450°F = 230°C   very hot oven
475°F = 245°C   very hot oven
500°F = 260°C   extremely hot oven/broiling
525°F = 275°C   extremely hot oven/broiling

LIQUID MEASURES CONVERSION

For foods such as yogurt, applesauce, or cottage cheese that are not quite liquid, but not quite solid, use fluid measures for conversion.

Both systems, the US Standard and Metric, use spoon measures. The sizes are slightly different, but the difference is not significant in general cooking (It may, however, be significant in baking.)

Tbs = tablespoon   teas = teaspoon

Spoons, cups, pints, quarts	Fluid oz	Milliliters (ml), deciliters (dl) and liters (l); rounded off
1 teas	⅙ oz	5 ml
3 teas (1 Tbs)	½ oz	15 ml

Spoons, cups, pints, quarts	Fluid oz	Milliliters (ml), deciliters (dl) and liters (l); rounded off
1 Tbs	1 oz	¼ dl (or 1 Tbs)
4 Tbs (¼ c)	2 oz	½ dl (or 4 Tbs)
⅓ c	2⅔ oz	¾ dl
½ c	4 oz	1 dl
¾ c	6 oz	1¾ dl
1 c	8 oz	250 ml (or ¼ L)
2 c (1 pint)	16 oz	500 ml (or ½ L)
4 c (1 quart)	32 oz	1 L
4 qt (1 gallon)	128 oz	3¾ L

SOLID MEASURES CONVERSION

Converting solid measures between US standard and metrics is not as straightforward as it might seem. The density of the substance being measured makes a big difference in the volume to weight conversion. For example, 1 tablespoon of flour is ¼ ounce and 8.75 grams whereas 1 tablespoon of butter or shortening is ½ ounce and 15 grams. The following chart is intended as a guide only, some experimentation may be necessary to achieve success.

Formulas for conversion
    ounces to grams: multiply ounces by 28.35
    grams to ounces: multiply grams figure by .035

ounces	pounds	grams	kilograms
1		30	
4	¼	115	
8	½	225	
9		250	¼
12	¾	430	
16	1	450	
18		500	½
	2¼	1000	1
	5		2¼
	10		4½

Linear Measures Conversion

Pan sizes are very different in countries that use metrics versus the US standard. This is more significant in baking than in general cooking.

Formulas for conversion
  inches to centimeters: multiply the inch by 2.54
  centimeters to inches: multiply the centimeter by 0.39

inches	cm	inches	cm
½	1½	9	23
1	2½	10	25
2	5	12 (1 ft.)	30
3	8	14	35
4	10	15	38½
5	13	16	40
6	15	18	45
7	18	20	50
8	20	24 (2 ft.)	60

Index